Medifocus Guidebook on:

Sjogren's Syndrome

Last Update: 16 January 2012

Medifocus.com, Inc.

11529 Daffodil Lane
Suite 200
Silver Spring, MD 20902

www.medifocus.com

(800) 965-3002

MediFocus Guide #RH011

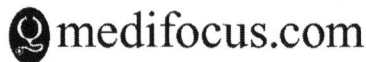

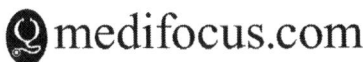

How To Use This Medifocus Guidebook

Before you start to review your *Guidebook*, it would be helpful to familiarize yourself with the organization and content of the information that is included in the Guidebook. Your *MediFocus Guidebook* is organized into the following five major sections.

- **Section 1: Background Information** - This section provides detailed information about the organization and content of the *Guidebook* including tips and suggestions for conducting additional research about the condition.

- **Section 2: The Intelligent Patient Overview** - This section is a comprehensive overview of the condition and includes important information about the cause of the disease, signs and symptoms, how the condition is diagnosed, the treatment options, quality of life issues, and questions to ask your doctor.

- **Section 3: Guide to the Medical Literature** - This section opens the door to the latest cutting-edge research and clinical advances recently published in leading medical journals. It consists of an extensive, focused selection of journal article references with links to the PubMed abstracts (summaries) of the articles. PubMed is the U.S. National Library of Medicine's database of references and abstracts from more than 4,500 medical and scientific articles published worldwide.

- **Section 4: Centers of Research** - This section is a unique directory of doctors, researchers, hospitals, medical centers, and research institutions with specialized interest and, in many cases, clinical expertise in the management of patients with the condition. You can use the "Centers of Research" directory to contact, consults, or network with leading experts in the field and to locate a hospital or medical center that can help you.

- **Section 5: Tips for Finding and Choosing a Doctor** - This section of your *Guidebook* offers important tips for how to find physicians as well as suggestions for how to make informed choices about choosing a doctor who is right for you.

- **Section 6: Directory of Organizations** - This section of your *Guidebook* is a directory of select disease organizations and support groups that are in the business of helping patients and their families by providing access to information, resources, and services. Many of these organizations can answer your questions, enable you to network with other patients, and help you find a doctor in your geographical area who specializes in managing your condition.

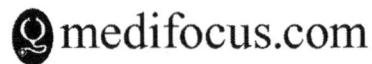

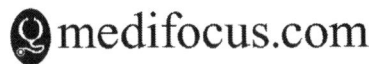

Disclaimer

Medifocus.com, Inc. serves only as a clearinghouse for medical health information and does not directly or indirectly practice medicine. Any information provided by *Medifocus.com, Inc.* is intended solely for educating our clients and should not be construed as medical advice or guidance, which should always be obtained from a licensed physician or other health-care professional. As such, the client assumes full responsibility for the appropriate use of the medical and health information contained in the Guidebook and agrees to hold *Medifocus.com, Inc.* and any of its third-party providers harmless from any and all claims or actions arising from the clients' use or reliance on the information contained in this Guidebook. Although *Medifocus.com, Inc.* makes every reasonable attempt to conduct a thorough search of the published medical literature, the possibility always exists that some significant articles may be missed.

Copyright

Copyright 2011, *Medifocus.com, Inc.* All rights reserved as to the selection, arrangement, formatting, and presentation of the information contained in this report, including our background and introductory information.

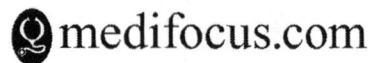

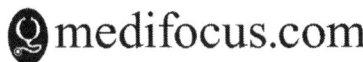

Table of Contents

Background Information 9
   Introduction 9
   About Your Medifocus Guidebook 11
   Ordering Full-Text Articles 15

The Intelligent Patient Overview 19

Guide to the Medical Literature 79
   Introduction 79
   Recent Literature: What Your Doctor Reads 81
      Review Articles 81
      General Interest Articles 94
      Drug Therapy Articles 123
      Clinical Trials Articles 126

Centers of Research 135
   United States 137
   Other Countries 145

Tips on Finding and Choosing a Doctor 165

Directory of Organizations 175

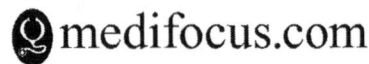

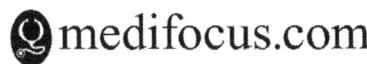

1 - Background Information

Introduction

Chronic or life-threatening illnesses can have a devastating impact on both the patient and the family. In today's new world of medicine, many consumers have come to realize that they are the ones who are primarily responsible for their own health care as well as for the health care of their loved ones.

When facing a chronic or life-threatening illness, you need to become an educated consumer in order to make an informed health care decision. Essentially that means finding out everything about the illness - the treatment options, the doctors, and the hospitals - so that you can become an educated health care consumer and make the tough decisions. In the past, consumers would go to a library and read everything available about a particular illness or medical condition. In today's world, many turn to the Internet for their medical information needs.

The first sites visited are usually the well known health "portals" or disease organizations and support groups which contain a general overview of the condition for the layperson. That's a good start but soon all of the basic information is exhausted and the need for more advanced information still exists. What are the latest "cutting-edge" treatment options? What are the results of the most up-to-date clinical trials? Who are the most notable experts? Where are the top-ranked medical institutions and hospitals?

The best source for authoritative medical information in the United States is the National Library of Medicine's medical database called PubMed, that indexes citations and abstracts (brief summaries) of over 7 million articles from more than 3,800 medical journals published worldwide. PubMed was developed for medical professionals and is the primary source utilized by health care providers for keeping up with the latest advances in clinical medicine.

A typical PubMed search for a specific disease or condition, however, usually retrieves hundreds or even thousands of "hits" of journal article citations. That's an avalanche of information that needs to be evaluated and transformed into truly useful knowledge. What are the most relevant journal articles? Which ones apply to your specific situation? Which articles are considered to be the most authoritative - the ones your physician would rely on in making clinical decisions? This is where *Medifocus.com* provides an effective solution.

Medifocus.com has developed an extensive library of *MediFocus Guidebooks* covering a wide spectrum of chronic and life threatening diseases. Each *MediFocus Guidebook* is a high quality, up- to-date digest of "professional-level" medical information consisting of the most relevant citations and abstracts of journal articles published in authoritative, trustworthy medical journals. This information represents the latest advances known to modern medicine for the treatment and management of the condition, including published results from clinical trials. Each *Guidebook* also includes a valuable index of leading authors and medical institutions as well as a directory of disease organizations and support groups. *MediFocus Guidebooks* are reviewed, revised and updated every 4-months to ensure that you receive the latest and most up-to-date information about the specific condition.

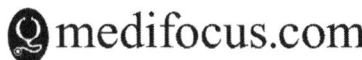

About Your MediFocus Guidebook

Introduction

Your *MediFocus Guidebook* is a valuable resource that represents a comprehensive synthesis of the most up-to-date, advanced medical information published about the condition in well-respected, trustworthy medical journals. It is the same type of professional-level information used by physicians and other health-care professionals to keep abreast of the latest developments in biomedical research and clinical medicine. The *Guidebook* is intended for patients who have a need for more advanced, in-depth medical information than is generally available to consumers from a variety of other resources. The primary goal of a *MediFocus Guidebook* is to educate patients and their families about their treatment options so that they can make informed health-care decisions and become active participants in the medical decision making process.

The *Guidebook* production process involves a team of experienced medical research professionals with vast experience in researching the published medical literature. This team approach to the development and production of the *MediFocus Guidebooks* is designed to ensure the accuracy, completeness, and clinical relevance of the information. The *Guidebook* is intended to serve as a basis for a more meaningful discussion between patients and their health-care providers in a joint effort to seek the most appropriate course of treatment for the disease.

Guidebook Organization and Content

Section 1 - Background Information
This section provides detailed information about the organization and content of the *Guidebook* including tips and suggestions for conducting additional research about the condition.

Section 2 - The Intelligent Patient Overview
This section of your *MediFocus Guidebook* represents a detailed overview of the disease or condition specifically written from the patient's perspective. It is designed to satisfy the basic informational needs of consumers and their families who are confronted with the illness and are facing difficult choices. Important aspects which are addressed in "The Intelligent Patient" section include:

- The etiology or cause of the disease
- Signs and symptoms
- How the condition is diagnosed

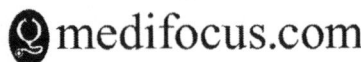

- The current standard of care for the disease
- Treatment options
- New developments
- Important questions to ask your health care provider

Section 3 - Guide to the Medical Literature

This is a roadmap to important and up-to-date medical literature published about the condition from authoritative, trustworthy medical journals. This is the same information that is used by physicians and researchers to keep up with the latest developments and breakthroughs in clinical medicine and biomedical research. A broad spectrum of articles is included in each *MediFocus Guidebook* to provide information about standard treatments, treatment options, new clinical developments, and advances in research. To facilitate your review and analysis of this information, the articles are grouped by specific categories. A typical *MediFocus Guidebook* usually contains one or more of the following article groupings:

- *Review Articles:* Articles included in this category are broad in scope and are intended to provide the reader with a detailed overview of the condition including such important aspects as its cause, diagnosis, treatment, and new advances.

- *General Interest Articles:* These articles are broad in scope and contain supplementary information about the condition that may be of interest to select groups of patients.

- *Drug Therapy:* Articles that provide information about the effectiveness of specific drugs or other biological agents for the treatment of the condition.

- *Surgical Therapy:* Articles that provide information about specific surgical treatments for the condition.

- *Clinical Trials:* Articles in this category summarize studies which compare the safety and efficacy of a new, experimental treatment modality to currently available standard treatments for the condition. In many cases, clinical trials represent the latest advances in the field and may be considered as being on the "cutting edge" of medicine. Some of these experimental treatments may have already been incorporated into clinical practice.

The following information is provided for each of the articles referenced in this section of your *MediFocus Guidebook:*

- Article title

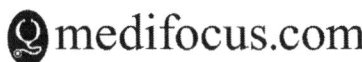

- Author Name(s)
- Institution where the study was done
- Journal reference (Volume, page numbers, year of publication)
- Link to Abstract (brief summary of the actual article)

Linking to Abstracts: Most of the medical journal articles referenced in this section of your *MediFocus Guidebook* include an abstract (brief summary of the actual article) that can be accessed online via the National Library of Medicine's PubMed® database. You can easily access the individual article abstracts online by entering the individual URL address for a particular article into your web browser, or by going to the URL listed on the bottom of each page of this section.

Section 4 - Centers of Research

We've compiled a unique directory of doctors, researchers, medical centers, and research institutions with specialized research interest, and in many cases, clinical expertise in the management of the specific medical condition. The "Centers of Research" directory is a valuable resource for quickly identifying and locating leading medical authorities and medical institutions within the United States and other countries that are considered to be at the forefront in clinical research and treatment of the condition.

Inclusion of the names of specific doctors, researchers, hospitals, medical centers, or research institutions in this *Guidebook* does not imply endorsement by Medifocus.com, Inc. or any of its affiliates. Consumers are encouraged to conduct additional research to identify health-care professionals, hospitals, and medical institutions with expertise in providing specific medical advice, guidance, and treatment for this condition.

Section 5 - Tips on Finding and Choosing a Doctor

One of the most important decisions confronting patients who have been diagnosed with a serious medical condition is finding and choosing a qualified physician who will deliver high-level, quality medical care in accordance with curently accepted guidelines and standards of care. Finding the "best" doctor to manage your condition, however, can be a frustrating and time-consuming experience unless you know what you are looking for and how to go about finding it. This section of your Guidebook offers important tips for how to find physicians as well as suggestions for how to make informed choices about choosing a doctor who is right for you.

Section 6 - Directory of Organizations

This section of your *Guidebook* is a directory of select disease organizations and support groups that are in the business of helping patients and their families by providing access to information, resources, and services. Many of these organizations can answer your questions, enable you to network with other patients, and help you find a doctor in your

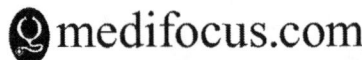

geographical area who specializes in managing your condition.

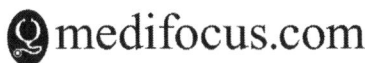

Ordering Full-Text Articles

After reviewing your *MediFocus Guidebook*, you may wish to order the full-text copy of some of the journal article citations that are referenced in the *Guidebook*. There are several options available for obtaining full-text copies of journal articles, however, with the exception of obtaining the article yourself by visiting a nearby medical library, most involve a fee to cover the costs of photocopying, delivering, and paying the copyright royalty fees set by the individual publishers of medical journals.

This section of your *MediFocus Guidebook* provides some basic information about how you can go about obtaining full-text copies of journal articles from various fee-based document delivery resources.

Commercial Document Delivery Services

There are numerous commercial document delivery companies that provide full-text photocopying and delivery services to the general public. The costs may vary from company to company so it is worth your while to carefully shop-around and compare prices. Some of these commercial document delivery services enable you to order articles directly online from the company's web site. You can locate companies that provide document delivery services by typing the key words "document delivery" into any major Internet search engine.

National Library of Medicine's "Loansome Doc" Document Retrieval Services

The National Library of Medicine (NLM), located in Bethesda, Maryland, offers full-text photocopying and delivery of journal articles through its on-line service known as "Loansome Doc". To learn more about how you can order articles using "Loansome Doc", please visit the NLM web site at:
http://www.nlm.nih.gov/pubs/factsheets/loansome_doc.html

Participating "Loansome Doc" Libraries: United States

In the United States there are approximately 250 medical libraries that participate in the National Library of Medicine's "Loansome Doc" document retrieval and delivery services for the general public. Please note that each participating library sets its own policies and

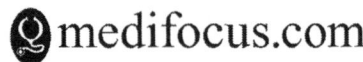

charges for providing document retrieval services. To order full-text copies of articles, simply contact a participating "Loansome Doc" medical library in your geographical area and ask to speak with one of the reference librarians. They can answer all of your questions including fees, delivery options, and turn-around time.

Here is how to find a participating "Loansome Doc" library in the U.S. that provides article retrieval services for the general public:

- **United States** - Contact a Regional Medical Library at 1-800-338-7657 (Monday - Friday; 8:30 AM - 5:30 PM). They will provide information about libraries in your area with which you may establish an account for the "Loansome Doc" service.

- **Canada** - Contact the Canada Institute for Scientific and Technical Information (CISTI) at 1-800-668-1222 for information about libraries in your area.

International MEDLARS Centers

If you reside outside the United States, you can obtain copies of medical journal articles through one of several participating International Medical Literature Analysis and Retrieval Systems (MEDLARS) Centers that provide "Loansome Doc" services in over 20 major countries. International MEDLARS Centers can be found in some of these countries: Australia, Canada, China, Egypt, France, Germany, Hong Kong, India, Israel, Italy, Japan, Korea, Kuwait, Mexico, Norway, Russia, South Africa, Sweden, and the United Kingdom. A complete listing of International MEDLARS Centers, including locations and telephone contact information can be viewed at:
http://www.nlm.nih.gov/pubs/factsheets/intlmedlars.html

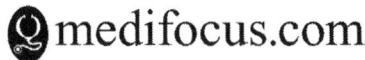

NOTES

Use this page for taking notes as you review your Guidebook

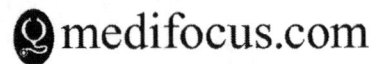

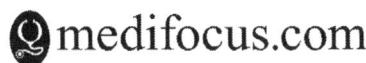

2 - The Intelligent Patient Overview

SJOGREN'S SYNDROME

Introduction to Sjogren's Syndrome

Most healthy people seldom give much thought to "automatic" physiological functions such as saliva production by our salivary glands or tear production by our lacrimal (tear) glands. We take for granted the fact that our salivary glands constantly produce the salivary fluids that keep our mouths moist and clean and that our lacrimal glands continuously produce a slow, steady flow of tears that lubricate our eyes to keep them comfortable and healthy. It is only when the normal physiological production of saliva and tears is disrupted, that we come to realize just how important a role these secretions play in our overall health and well-being.

Sjogren's syndrome is a chronic, slowly progressive, inflammatory autoimmune disorder characterized by the infiltration of specialized cells of the immune system called *lymphocytes* (T-cells in the majority of cases), *monocytes*, and *plasma cells* into the *parotid* (salivary) glands and *lacrimal* (tear) glands. These glands are part of a group of *exocrine glands* whose secretions pass into a system of ducts that lead ultimately to the exterior of the body. This chronic lymphocytic infiltration interferes with the normal function of these glands and eventually results in a significant reduction or cessation in the production and secretion of saliva and tears. The condition is named after Henry Sjogren, a Swedish ophthalmologist, who first described the primary clinical features of this disorder in 1933.

Two distinct forms of Sjogren's syndrome have been recognized:

- *Primary* Sjogren's syndrome - defined as dry eye and dry mouth that occurs by itself and is not associated with another autoimmune disorder. Primary Sjogren's syndrome occurs in approximately 50% of cases according to the Sjogren's Foundation of America.
- *Secondary* Sjogren's syndrome - characterized by dry eye and dry mouth that occurs in the presence of a major underlying *autoimmune connective tissue disease* such as rheumatoid arthritis, systemic lupus erythematosus, or scleroderma.

Sjogren's syndrome is difficult to diagnose since it is comprised of a wide range of symptoms that may not appear concurrently and, as a result, often are treated as individual

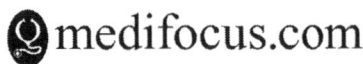

conditions rather than as a total syndrome. Alternatively, diagnosis may be missed since the individual symptoms of Sjogren's syndrome mimic symptoms related to many other medical conditions. Some studies indicate that many patients with Sjogren's syndrome may suffer for an average of 10 years before they are correctly diagnosed.

While Sjogren's syndrome is a chronic, progressive condition, the progression for most patients is very slow. Sjogren's syndrome is more benign than other autoimmune diseases and typically is not associated with rapid deterioration of symptoms or dramatic changes in condition. Sjogren's syndrome is considered to be more a condition of morbidity (on-going illness) rather than mortality. The most serious aspect of Sjogren's syndrome, however, is the increased risk (6.5-fold) of developing non-Hodgkin's lymphoma which is approximately 44 times greater than the risk of the general population, and a 1000-fold increased risk of parotid gland marginal zone lymphoma, and diffuse large B-cell and follicular lymphomas. The risk of lymphomas is closely related to B-cell hyperreactivity.

Major Characteristics of Sjogren's Disease

The clinical manifestations of Sjogren's syndrome include:

- Dry mouth (*xerostomia*) - caused by reduced saliva production
- Dry eyes (*xerophthalmia*) - caused by reduced production of tears by the lacrimal glands, also called *keratoconjunctiva sicca*
- Exraglandular manifestations

Dryness in Sjogren's syndrome is not generally due to the destruction of the salivary and lacrimal glands. Most biopsy reports show that there is a remnant of the gland but that the tissue in that remnant is inflamed and dysfunctional apparently due to substances that are released in the inflammatory process. This causes a loss of viscosity which increases the friction in areas that the saliva and tears should be lubricating. As a result of the increased friction, the patient experiences chronic inflammation, abrasions of the cornea, (caused by lack of tears), and severe dental problems (caused by lack of saliva).

Dry Mouth in Sjogren's Syndrome

Three pairs of bilateral salivary glands (one pair on each side of the face) are responsible for the production of 90% of the approximately 1.5 liters of saliva that we produce daily. These glands are:

- Parotid glands - these glands are located in front of the ears and extend downward to beneath the earlobes along the border of the lower jaw. They produce up to 70% of the saliva as a result of stimulation (i.e., chewing or eating). This is known as *stimulated saliva*.

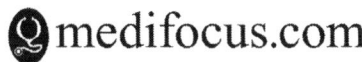

- Submandibular glands (also called *submaxillary*) - these walnut sized glands are located under the lower jaw. These glands produce up to 80% of the saliva at rest, also called *unstimulated saliva*.
- Sublingual glands - these glands are located beneath the floor of the tongue and also contribute to saliva production.

There are also many tiny salivary glands located in the lips, inner cheek area, and other linings in the mouth and throat that produce the remaining 10% of our saliva.

Role of Saliva
Normal salivary function originates in specialized glandular cells called *muscarinic M3 receptor cells* and when they are stimulated, saliva is produced. Saliva is a clear watery fluid which is slightly viscous and originates in the salivary glands. The primary component is water (up to 98%) and the remainder is a combination of enzymes, proteins, antibodies, and other substances that perform many important functions including:

- Cleansing and lubricating the oral cavity
- Initiating the breakdown of food for digestion
- Facilitating eating (chewing, swallowing)
- Improving taste
- Removing food debris from the mouth
- Preventing growth and development of viral, bacterial, and fungal infection (anti-microbial protection)
- Controlling the pH level (acid) in the mouth which reduces the development of dental cavities
- Facilitating speech
- Protecting the health of the tongue

Patients with Sjogren's syndrome who suffer from dry mouth may have several oral-related problems, many of which are described below.

Dry Eyes in Sjogren's Syndrome

The primary function of tears is to bathe and cleanse the eye, keep it free from dust, and assist in lubrication so that it turns easily in its socket. Tears are produced by the lacrimal glands, which are located above the outer corners of each eye. Blinking wipes away the tears by collecting it at the inner corner of the eye, where it is carried away via the tear ducts.

Tears are comprised of water as well as other components that protect the surface of the eyes. They contain many elements vital to the health of the eye surface such as epithelial growth factor (regulates cell growth and other functions), fibronectin (protein that supports cellular function), and vitamins. They also contain anti-microbial agents and nourishing

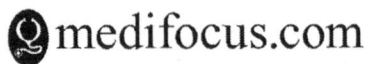

substances that help in the mechanical and optical functioning of the eye.

Patients with Sjogren's syndrome who suffer from dry eye can develop severe ocular disorders in the absence of sufficient tears including dry, itchy, irritated and/or red eyes. Patients frequently report *photophobia* (aversion to light) and increased ocular irritation, especially at night. See the Guidebook section called *Signs and Symptoms* for further details.

Collectively, dry mouth and dry eyes are the two primary symptoms of Sjogren's syndrome and are known as the *sicca (dry) syndrome*.

Extraglandular Involvement in Sjogren's Disease

In approximately 40% of patients, Sjogren's syndrome progresses beyond the exocrine glands and systemic (*extraglandular*) features develop. In addition to dry mouth and dry eyes, these patients also develop a more systemic form of Sjogren's with the involvement of other organ systems (extraglandular). Symptoms include:

- Cutaneous symptoms - Skin involvement is the most common systemic manifestation of Sjogren's syndrome. Symptoms may include:

  - rash
  - itching
  - purpura (the purple color of skin after blood has "leaked" under it)
  - vasculitis (inflammation of the blood vessels)

- Musculoskeletal symptoms such as painful joints

- Pulmonary symptoms such as a dry cough
- Hematological symptoms such as *cytopenia* (reduction in the number of cells circulating in the blood)
- Lymphoproliferative disorders such as *lymphoma* (cancer that starts in the cells of the immune system)

Incidence of Sjogren's Syndrome

It has been estimated that up to 4 million Americans are afflicted with Sjogren's syndrome and that 1-2% of the population in the United States has been diagnosed with Sjogren's syndrome. However, because the disorder may be difficult to diagnose, the incidence of the disease may be considerably higher. Sjogren's syndrome is a condition that affects primarily women with a female to male ratio of about 24:1, meaning that about 95% of people who suffer from Sjogren's syndrome are women. Symptoms of the disorder most

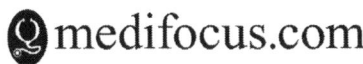

often begin between the ages of 40-60, predominantly in peri/post menopausal women, but are also seen in young women in their 20s and 30s. The average age of onset is 52 years old. The overall prevalence of Sjogren's syndrome in the general population has been estimated to range from 0.5% to 3.0%.

Systemic lupus erythematosus (SLE) shares many features with Sjogren's syndrome and it is believed that a subset of peri/post menopausal women diagnosed with SLE may actually have Sjogren's syndrome. Approximately 30% of patients with rheumatoid arthritis and SLE also suffer from Sjogren's syndrome. In fact, it has been estimated that 50-60% of the cases of Sjogren's syndrome are secondary to another underlying autoimmune disorder such as rheumatoid arthritis, systemic sclerosis (scleroderma), or SLE.

Causes of Sjogren's Syndrome

Sjogren's syndrome is an autoimmune condition marked by the presence of antinuclear antibodies and rheumatoid factor. Other antibodies (anti-Ro) are associated with extraglandular (outside of the glands) manifestations of Sjogren's syndrome. Organ-specific antibodies are found in approximately 60% of patients with Sjogren's syndrome.

Sjogren's syndrome is associated with chronic stimulation of the immune system, specifically B-cells and T-cells. Histologically (microscopic anatomy of the cells), focal lymphocytic infiltrates (a collection of fluid and cells in the tissue) are located mostly around glandular ducts (salivary and lacrimal ducts) and other exocrine glands (skin, lungs, gastrointestinal tract, and vagina). The infiltrate contains plasma cells, T-cells in most cases, and B-cells in some cases. Eventually, the infiltrate grows and occupies the inner epithelium (inner lining of the gland) that leads to dysfunction and enlargement of the gland as well as degeneration, necrosis, and atrophy.

Although the exact cause of Sjogren's syndrome remains unknown, several theories have been proposed in an attempt to explain the pathophysiology of the disorder. These include:

- Chronic inflammation
- Cellular apoptosis
- Autonomic dysfunction
- Genetic predisposition
- Neurotransmitter abnormality
- Autoimmune response to a viral trigger

Chronic Inflammation Theory
The chronic inflammation theory proposes that Sjogren's syndrome is caused by the

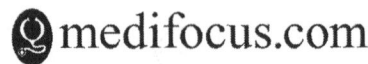

continuous infiltration of immune cells (lymphocytes, monocytes, and plasma cells) into the salivary and lacrimal glands, which eventually results in replacement of normal glandular tissue with chronic inflammatory cells, causing progressive dysfunction of the glands with reduced production and secretion of saliva and tears.

Evidence shows that defective glandular tissue seems to be inherently related to the development of antigens which, for unknown reasons, instead of being seen as part of the body, become the focus of an autoimmune attack, bringing on the continued infiltration of lymphocytes. In addition, the attacking cells (B/T-lymphocytes) fail to undergo normal apoptosis (cell death) which results in their proliferation and which may be a factor in prolonging the autoimmune process.

Cellular Apoptosis Theory

The term "apoptosis" refers to death of a cell and is a form of cellular "self-destruction". It has been hypothesized that apoptosis of glandular cells, especially ductal cells, may eventually lead to the glandular dysfunction that is responsible for the classic dry eye and dry mouth symptoms of Sjogren's syndrome. Apoptosis of glandular cells may be triggered by viral infections including:

- Epstein-Barr virus (EBV) infection
- Hepatitis C virus (HCV) infection
- Human Immunodeficiency Virus (HIV) infection

Autonomic Dysfunction Theory

This theory proposes that a dysfunction of the *autonomic nervous system*, the part of the nervous system that controls the production and secretion of saliva and tears, may be a major contributing factor leading to glandular dysfunction and the development of Sjogren's syndrome.

Genetic Predisposition Theory

Proponents of this theory believe that some people who develop Sjogren's syndrome may be genetically predisposed to this disorder. Evidence supporting a genetic predisposition for Sjogren's syndrome has been linked to the *major histocompatibility complex* genes known as *human leukocyte antigens* (HLAs). An increased prevalence of specific HLA genes, including HLAB8, DR3, and DRw52, has been found in patients with primary Sjogren's syndrome.

Genetic evidence has also recently indicated that defective glandular development may predispose an individual to developing epithelial glandular cells that secrete certain immuno-stimulatory agents which are not seen in patients who do not have Sjogren's syndrome.

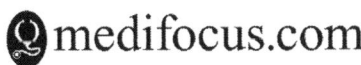

Neurotransmitter Abnormality

Biopsies of the salivary glands of patients with Sjogren's syndrome have shown that while only 50-60% of glandular tissue is destroyed, the symptoms of dry mouth and dry eye are as severe as if only minimal healthy tissue remained. This puzzle has led some scientists to theorize that some aspect of the immune cells that are produced impair the release of the neurotransmitter acetylcholine and that this may account for the cessation or severe reduction of saliva or tear production, even in the presence of healthy glandular tissue.

Autoimmune Response to a Viral Trigger

Another theory proposes that a trigger, such as a viral infection, may induce an autoimmune T-cell response leading to chronic destruction of epithelial cells, production of inflammatory cells, and the release of chemicals (cytokines, chemokynes) that further stimulate the production of T- and B-cells with the release of autoantibodies. In a subset of these cases, certain B-cell-related factors in the inflamed salivary glands stimulate further production of B-cells which elevates the risk for lymphoma.

Excessive B-cell activation is responsible for many of the extraglandular manifestations of primary Sjogren's syndrome including arthritis, vasculitis, neuropathy, and others. To read more about the role of B-cells in Sjogren's syndrome, please click on the following link: http://www.ncbi.nlm.nih.gov/pubmed/19758218

Signs and Symptoms of Sjogren's Syndrome

The signs and symptoms of Sjogren's syndrome may be grouped as follows:

- Oral manifestations
- Ocular manifestations
- Systemic manifestations

Oral Manifestations

The major oral manifestation of Sjogren's syndrome is dry mouth (*xerostomia*) resulting in a parched, dry sensation in the mouth and throat. It has been reported that approximately 94% of patients with Sjogren's syndrome experience dry mouth.

Swallowing flushes out the mouth by clearing the oral cavity of saliva, food debris and microorganisms. When this process is interrupted, as occurs in Sjogren's syndrome, there is an increase in many types of microorganisms in the mouth which leads to dental caries (cavities), periodontal disease, and infection.

The mouth may appear moist in the early stages of Sjogren's syndrome, but as the disease progresses, the dryness becomes more pronounced as saliva ceases to pool at the bottom of the mouth and extreme dryness sets in. This may cause the tongue to stick to the roof of the mouth and as a result affects speech clarity and/or may cause a clicking dimension to speech. Erythema (redness), fissures, and ulcerations may develop with continued dryness.

Other oral manifestations of the disorder may include:

- Tongue

    - dry, red, or painful tongue (*glossodynia*)
    - ulcers on the tongue
    - impaired taste bud function
    - atrophic changes (wasting or diminution) of the taste buds
    - tongue to palate adhesion affecting speaking and eating

- Eating function

    - difficulty chewing and swallowing food, especially dry, crumbly foods such as crackers
    - changes in the ability to taste food (*dysgeusia*)
    - food adhesion to dental surfaces

- Oral mucosa

    - fungal infections such as *chronic erythematous candidiasis* (causes red patches and thinning of mucosa on the palate and inner lining of the cheeks and lips) may affect up to 30% of patients
    - cracked lips with fissures (*cheilitis*)
    - *angular cheilitis* - a painful cracking and soreness that develops at the corners of the mouth
    - fissures of the inner tissue lining the mouth and cheek

- Oral cavity

    - severe dryness
    - burning or tingling sensation in the mouth or soreness
    - unpleasant taste in the mouth
    - halitosis (bad breath)
    - tooth decay -first appears at the gum margins, progressing further into the mouth over time and affects about 70% of Sjogren's patients
    - cavities
    - difficulty anchoring dentures in the gums

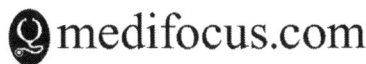

- gum sores due to dentures
- voice alterations (hoarseness or coarse voice)

- Swelling of the salivary glands (particularly the parotid gland) - this occurs in approximately one third of patients with primary Sjogren's syndrome. It may begin on one side only and develop into bilateral swelling. The enlargement may be chronic or episodic and leads to loss of function of the gland which results in a further decrease of salivary production and flow rates.

Ocular Manifestations

The most common ocular feature of Sjogren's syndrome is dry eye, also known as *xerophthalmia* and *keratoconjunctivitis sicca* (KCS). Approximately 65% of patients diagnosed with Sjogren's syndrome complain of dry eyes.

Other ocular manifestations of Sjogren's syndrome include:

- Redness, soreness, burning, or itching eyes
- Foreign body sensation in eyes - sometimes described as "grains of sand in eyes"
- Difficulty tolerating contact lenses
- Photophobia - avoidance of light
- Eye fatigue - particularly when reading or watching television
- Discharge or secretions from the eyes due to abnormal mucus production
- Feeling a film or lack of acuity in the visual field
- Corneal ulceration
- Blurred vision

Some patients have reported that ocular symptoms associated with Sjogren's syndrome are often exacerbated by:

- Low humidity
- Dry climate
- Exposure to cigarette smoke
- Anticholinergic drugs (a class of drugs that block a neurotransmitter called *acetylcholine*)

Systemic Manifestations
Sinus Symptoms
Nasal or sinus symptoms are attributable to Sjogren's syndrome in up to 50% of patients who experience atrophy of the mucus lining of the nose. Symptoms include:

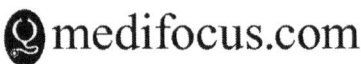

- Nasal crusting
- Epistaxis (nose bleeds)
- Perforation of the septum
- Hyposmia (diminished sensitivity to smell)
- Hypogeusia (diminished sensitivity to taste)

Musculoskeletal Symptoms

Approximately 55% of patients with primary Sjogren's syndrome experience musculoskeletal symptoms including:

- Arthralgia (non-inflammatory joint pain) or arthropathy (diseases of the joint) that occurs in up to 50% of patients
- Arthritis (inflammatory joint pain) is thought to occur in at least 30% of patients and tends to be relapsing, remitting, and tends to occur symmetrically on the right and left sides. Some patients exhibit signs of arthritis 5-10 years before they are diagnosed with Sjogren's syndrome.
- Myositis - inflammation of muscle tissue
- Myalgia (general term for noninflammatory muscular pain) - up to 20% of patients with Sjogren's syndrome suffer from fibromyalgia
- Muscle weakness

Fatigue

One of the most debilitating systemic features of Sjogren's syndrome is fatigue which many individuals with Sjogren's syndrome describe as more distressing than any other symptom. Fatigue occurs in approximately 50-70% of patients with Sjogren's syndrome.

Sleep disorders are also common in patients with Sjogren's syndrome, which may be a factor in fatigue. Patients report that they sleep but do not feel well-rested when they wake up. Some clinicians are of the opinion that the excessive fatigue experienced by these patients may be related to subclinical hypothyroidism which is also associated with Sjogren's syndrome.

Cutaneous Symptoms

Estimates of the percentage of Sjogren's syndrome patients who experience skin problems range from 10-40%. *Cutaneous vasculitis* (inflammation of the blood vessels in the skin) is one of the most characteristic extraglandular manifestations of Sjogren's syndrome and is thought to be due to lymphocytic infiltration into the walls of the blood vessels. Typically, small blood vessels are affected more than large ones.

The most common forms of cutaneous vasculitis seen in Sjogren's syndrome patients (typically patients who have anti-Ro and anti-La antibodies) are:

- Palpable or nonpalpable *purpura* (purple spots on the skin after blood "leaks" underneath, similar to a bruise) which can cause raised, red skin lesions
- Urticarial lesions (hives)
- Erythematosus micropapules (red spots)

Patients with cutaneous vasculitis also may develop non-vasculitic lesions including:

- *Petechiae* - pinpoint dots
- *Photosensitive cutaneous lesions* - light-sensitive lesions (also seen in patients with systemic lupus erythematosus)
- *Livedo reticularis* - marbled appearance of the skin
- *Lichen planus* - small, itchy pink or purple spots on arm and/or legs
- *Thrombocytopenic purpura* - purple areas on the skin related to a decrease in blood platelets
- *Vitiligo* - white patches on skin due to loss of pigmentation

Cutaneous vasculitis (as well as other forms of vasculitis - see below) is considered to be a significant prognostic indicator with the development of lymphoma and mortality. A large 2004 study of 558 Sjogren's syndrome patients diagnosed with cutaneous involvement reported that 58% of the patients had cutaneous vasculitis and showed a higher incidence of:

- Peripheral neuropathy - damage to the nerves that supply the arms and legs characterized by burning, tingling, numbness and pain
- Raynaud's phenomenon - a circulatory disorder caused by insufficient blood supply to the hands and feet
- Renal (kidney) involvement
- Presence of autoimmune markers such as antinuclear antibodies (ANA) and rheumatoid factor
- B-cell lymphoma

Other skin problems that may be experienced by patients with Sjogren's syndrome include:

- Dry skin (*xerosis*) - affects up to 55% of patients with Sjogren's syndrome
- Itchy skin
- Burning skin - may be experienced in up to 20% of patients with Sjogren's syndrome
- Skin rashes - may be experienced in up to 10% of patients with Sjogren's syndrome
- Raynaud's phenomenon - may appear many years before the development of symptoms of dry mouth and dry eyes. Estimated to occur in up to 30% of patients, it is usually of minor clinical significance.

Vasculitis

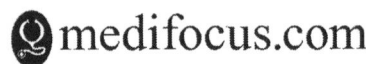

Vasculitis in general refers to inflammation of the blood vessels and is estimated to occur in up to 10% of patients with Sjogren's syndrome. It typically involves small- and medium-blood vessels and ranges from benign (most common) to life-threatening (rare). Risk factors for development of vasculitis include:

- Parotid scintigraphy - Grades III-IV (a diagnostic technique based on the detection of radiation emitted by radioactive substances injected into the body; also called radionuclide scanning), considered an independent prognostic factor of development of vasculitis.
- Low C3 and/or C4 levels in the blood (*hypocomplementemia*).
- *Cryoglobulinemia* (low levels of immunoglobulins that congeal in cold temperatures)
- Anti Ro/La antibodies.

Life-threatening vasculitis, however, is rare and appears to be related to elevated levels of cryoglobulins (abnormal blood proteins) in the blood plasma (*cryoglobulinemia*).

Pulmonary Symptoms

The most common pulmonary (lung) symptom of Sjogren's syndrome is a dry cough due to xerotrachea (dry, scratchy trachea). Estimates of pulmonary involvement vary widely in the literature and ranges from 9-75% of patients with Sjogren's syndrome (depending upon the diagnostic techniques used) but it is rarely clinically significant. Evidence of pulmonary changes appears on up to 50% of lung scans by some estimates, but they usually remain subclinical (without obvious symptoms). Progression is very slow and typically does not develop into clinically significant pulmonary disease. In one study examining the incidence of pulmonary involvement in patients with Sjogren's syndrome, approximately 87% of patients had some degree abnormal pulmonary function.

Recent studies show that pulmonary involvement is typically at the bronchial or bronchiolar level, but interstitial disease (damage to lung tissue) can occur. Other pulmonary complications which may occur include:

- *Tracheobronchia sicca* - dryness of the tracheal pathways leading to continual dry cough
- *Lymphocytic interstitial pneumonitis* - a syndrome characterized by fever, cough, and shortness of breath with infiltrates of dense interstitial accumulations of lymphocytes and plasma cells
- *Pulmonary pseudolymphoma* - a benign accumulation of inflammatory lymphoid cells in the lung
- *Alveolitis* - inflammation of the air sacs (alveoli) in the lungs where the exchange of oxygen and carbon dioxide takes place
- Various types of pneumonia, such as *nonspecific interstitial pneumonia*, *organizing pneumonia* (noninfectious inflammation of the bronchioles and surrounding lung

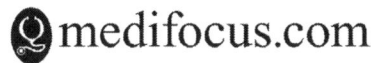

tissue), or *usual interstitial pneumonia* (changes in lung tissue indicative of fibrosis or scarring)
- Primary lymphoma of the lung
- Mucosa associated lymphoid tissue (MALT)
- Lung hypersensitivity
- Diffuse interstitial amyloidosis (deposit or accumulation of protein in lung tissue) - not a common development but associated with progressive deterioration and a poor prognosis.

Tracheobronchial sicca and interstitial pneumonitis are the most common lung conditions associated with Sjogren's syndrome.

To read more about interstitial lung disease in primary Sjogren's syndrome, please click on the following link: http://www.ncbi.nlm.nih.gov/pubmed/19390161

Kidney/Bladder Symptoms

Kidney and other genitourinary symptoms are thought to occur in approximately 10% of patients with primary Sjogren's syndrome and are caused by the infiltration of lymphocytes into the kidneys. Clinically significant renal involvement is rare.

Renal conditions which may develop in patients with Sjogren's syndrome, include:

- *Chronic interstitial cystitis* - a chronic, inflammatory condition of the bladder wall that is a common condition among patients with Sjogren's syndrome. Recent studies have found that many people with Sjogren's syndrome also suffer from chronic interstitial cystitis in the absence of bacterial infection. The symptoms are similar to those of a urinary tract infection; however, urine cultures are negative. The diagnosis is confirmed by cystoscopy and biopsy.
- Tubular disease such as *tubulointerstitial nephritis* - an inflammation of the tubules of the kidney and the spaces between the tubules and the glomeruli (renal capillaries). Tubular involvement is usually found in younger patients and typically remains subclinical without developing into renal failure.
- *Renal tubular acidosis* develops when the kidneys fail to excrete acids into the urine resulting in a build-up of acids in the bloodstream. Without proper treatment, this condition can lead to a variety of other complications including kidney stones and progressive kidney failure.
- Glomerular diseases such as *membranous glomerulonephritis* - an inflammation of the glomeruli of the kidneys caused by the accumulation of protein in the bloodstream (proteinuria). Glomerular involvement is a severe manifestation of extraglandular disease involvement of Sjogren's syndrome. It typically appears later in the course of Sjogren's syndrome and is associated with morbidity and mortality. Early diagnosis and treatment is very important.

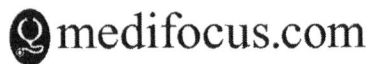

- *Renal calculi* - kidney stones
- Deterioration of renal function due to certain medications given to treat Sjogren's syndrome such as non-steroidal anti-inflammatory drugs.

Gastrointestinal Symptoms

Saliva plays a major role in the initial phases of digestion and reduced amounts or absence of saliva can cause a disruption in the normal function of the gastrointestinal tract. Esophageal dryness is the most common gastrointestinal manifestation of Sjogren's syndrome and is the cause of dysphagia (difficulty swallowing) experienced by many people with Sjogren's syndrome. Other difficulties which patients may experience include:

- Regurgitation of food
- Reflux of gastric acid into the esophagus (neutralizing properties of saliva are lacking)
- Nausea
- Epigastric pain
- Gastritis - irritation of the stomach lining that causes "heartburn"
- Celiac sprue - sensitivity to gluten causing impaired food absorption
- Presence of *Helicobacter pylori* which is associated with MALT lymphoma
- Gastrotracheal reflux - gastric acid refluxes not just to the esophagus but up to the trachea. Continual reflux can lead to abnormal changes in tracheal tissue.

Development of pancreatitis is rare in patients with Sjogren's syndrome; however, laboratory studies may show elevated levels of certain gastric enzymes (e.g., gastrin) and biopsy may show infiltration of lymphocytes into the gastric mucosa.

Neurologic Symptoms

Approximately 10%-30% of Sjogren's patients (some estimates are as high as 60%) develop neurological symptoms including:

- *Polyneuropathy* - pure or predominantly sensory polyneuropathies cause pain, numbness, tingling, and muscle weakness in the hands, arms, feel, and legs (this is the most common neurologic manifestations of SS)
- *Cranial neuropathy* - most often affecting the trigeminal nerve; may cause a condition called trigeminal neuralgia (intense, sharp pain in the area of the face).
- *Transverse myelitis* - an acute spinal cord disorder causing sudden low back pain, muscle weakness, and abnormal sensations in the lower extremities. This is one of several sclerosis-like syndromes that may occur in a minority (up to 1%) of patients with Sjogren's syndrome.
- Abnormal nerve conduction
- Motor neuropathy
- Demyelinating neuropathy (neuropathy caused by the destruction of myelin that

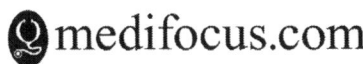

surrounds the sheath of the nerve cell)
- Myelopathy (conditions affecting the spinal cord)
- Loss of small-diameter nerve fibers

It is sometimes difficult to differentiate between age-related and Sjogren's syndrome-related neurological symptoms, since there is considerable overlap between them. Also, the most common age of onset of Sjogren's syndrome is at a time in life when common aging changes may occur naturally. Thus information is limited regarding specific neurologic symptoms in elderly patients with Sjogren's syndrome.

Gynecologic Symptoms

The most common gynecological manifestation of Sjogren's syndrome in women is vaginal dryness which leads to significant general discomfort. It has been estimated that up to 25% of women with Sjogren's syndrome complain of vaginal symptoms but fertility and childbirth do not appear to be affected by the presence of Sjogren's syndrome. *Dyspareunia*, painful intercourse, is thought to affect approximately 40% of premenopausal women and is secondary to insufficient lubrication of the vaginal region.

When vaginal dryness develops, it should be treated promptly because it can cause:

- Uncomfortable vaginal itching
- Difficulty in urination
- Urinary tract infections
- Yeast infections

It is thought that vaginal lubrication involves fluid from the bloodstream and from the cervical mucosa that flow through the vaginal wall, and is not related to fluid produced by local glands. When women develop Sjogren's syndrome, lymphocytic inflammatory cells infiltrate the vascular system supplying fluid to the vagina, thereby causing a reduction in vaginal lubrication.

Hematologic Abnormalities

Hematologic (blood-related) abnormalities in Sjogren's syndrome are usually asymptomatic and include:

- Elevated sedimentation rate - this is reported in the blood of up to 70% of patients with Sjogren's syndrome.
- Anemia - the number of red blood cells in the bloodstream is lower than normal
- Leukopenia - the number of white blood cells (leukocytes) in the bloodstream is lower than normal
- Autoimmune cytopenia (reduced number of cells circulating in the blood) - this is usually a mild condition but can develop into a serious condition

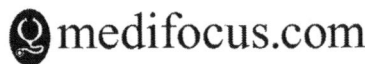

- Hyper/hypoglobulinemia (elevated or reduced levels of globulins in the blood)

Lymphoproliferative Disease

Lymphoma develops in approximately 5% of patients diagnosed with Sjogren's syndrome. It has been estimated that patients with primary and secondary Sjogren's syndrome have an approximately 44-fold increased risk for developing lymphoma as compared with healthy, age-matched controls. The most common form of lymphoma associated with Sjogren's syndrome is low or intermediate grade B-cell lymphoma that originates in mucosa-associated lymphoid tissue. Lymphoma occurs more frequently in patients with primary Sjogren's syndrome than secondary Sjogren's syndrome.

It is thought that the chronic stimulation and proliferation of monoclonal B cells in Sjogren's syndrome is related to the transition that takes place from an autoimmune status to the development of non-Hodgkin's lymphoma. Most lymphomas associated with Sjogren's syndrome are characterized as:

- Low- or intermediate-grade malignancy potential
- Localized in extranodal spaces (spaces around the outside of the lymph nodes)

Clinical or laboratory evidence of an emerging lymphoma may include:

- Persistent enlargement of parotid (salivary) glands
- Persistent enlargement of the spleen (splenomegaly)
- Persistent enlargement of lymph nodes (lymphadenopathy)
- Type II mixed monoclonal cryoglobulinemia
- Low levels of complement factors C3 or C4 in the bloodstream
- Inflammation of the blood vessels (vasculitis)

Other lymph-related conditions that may develop with Sjogren's syndrome include:

- Lymphopenia - reduced circulating lymphocytes in the bloodstream
- Waldenstrom's macroglobulinemia - cancer of the B-lymphocytes (a type of white blood cell) which causes overproduction of monoclonal macroglobulins (IgM antibody)
- Lymphadenopathy - enlargement of the lymph glands

Cardiac Symptoms

Cardiac conditions which may be associated with Sjogren's syndrome include:

- Pericarditis - inflammation of the sac surrounding the heart
- Pulmonary hypertension - high blood pressure in the arteries that supply the lungs
- Orthostatic hypotension - abnormal and sudden changes in blood pressure when

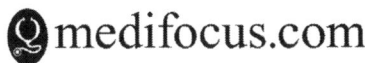

changing from sitting or lying to standing).

Hepatobiliary Symptoms
Some patients may also develop hepatitis C or a condition called *primary biliary cirrhosis*, a liver disease that slowly destroys the bile ducts and leads to the build-up of bile in the liver and eventual cirrhosis (hardening) of the liver. Typically, however, liver involvement in patients with Sjogren's syndrome is rare (up to 5% of Sjogren's syndrome patients) and when it does occur, it is usually asymptomatic and subclinical (disease has not yet exhibited overt symptoms).

Psychiatric Symptoms
The most common psychiatric conditions associated with Sjogren's syndrome are:

- Depression
- Anxiety

The high incidence of these conditions has led some researchers to believe that they may be part of Sjogren's syndrome rather than a reaction to the stress. Depression and anxiety also commonly precede the diagnosis of systemic lupus erythematosus as well as other autoimmune conditions. Other symptoms that may develop include subtle changes in cognitive function, memory, and concentration.

Thyroid Symptoms
Antibodies directed to the thyroid gland can be detected in approximately 50% of people diagnosed with Sjogren's syndrome, while only half of these patients demonstrate abnormalities on thyroid function tests. Various thyroid abnormalities, including *Hashimoto's thyroiditis* (a type of autoimmune thyroid disease) and hypothyroidism (low thyroid function) have been associated with Sjogren's syndrome. It is estimated that approximately 10% of patients with autoimmune thyroid disease may have Sjogren's syndrome.

To read more about thyroid disease and Sjogren's syndrome, please click on the following link: http://www.ncbi.nlm.nih.gov/pubmed/17558463

Laryngeal Symptoms
Lesions of the vocal cords have been associated with Sjogren's syndrome and can cause hoarseness, which in rare cases may be the first indication of Sjogren's syndrome. Conditions associated with these lesions include:

- Bamboo node - an unusual white or yellow transverse lesion typically located in the middle third of the vocal cord, and most frequently associated with autoimmune diseases.

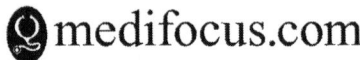

- Vocal cord nodules

Otologic Symptoms
Some patients with Sjogren's syndrome demonstrate a mild to moderate sensorineural hearing loss of high frequency sounds. The connection to Sjogren's syndrome pathology is not well understood.

Diagnosis of Sjogren's Syndrome

As with other autoimmune disorders, the symptoms of Sjogren's syndrome develop slowly over time. Due to the slow progression of symptoms, there is typically up to a 10-year gap between the onset of symptoms and diagnosis of the disorder. Also, because of the typical age range of onset of Sjogren's syndrome (middle-age women), some symptoms of Sjogren's syndrome can be confused with symptoms often seen with normal aging (e.g., vaginal dryness) of menopausal women which can delay the accurate diagnosis of Sjogren's syndrome.

Diagnosis of Sjogren's syndrome is often difficult to establish with people who present with less definitive symptoms or borderline antibody values. In addition, sicca symptoms, namely dry eyes and dry mouth, can be present with many other medical conditions that add to the difficulty in identifying primary Sjogren's syndrome.

Early and accurate diagnosis of Sjogren's syndrome is important because initiation of appropriate therapy can prevent further damage. For example:

- Treating the symptoms of dry mouth can reduce oral problems such as cavities, periodontal diseases, oral infections
- Treating the symptoms of dry eyes can minimize ocular damage
- Earlier diagnosis and initiation of treatment for systemic complications of Sjogren's syndrome can improve prognosis (chance of recovery)

There is no single diagnostic test available for Sjogren's syndrome. Rather, a thorough medical history, a review of signs and symptoms, a physical examination, and select diagnostic and laboratory tests are used to establish the diagnosis. In many cases, patients are referred to several medical specialists (e.g., rheumatologist, ophthalmologist, and dentist) who, by working together, are able to link the pieces of the puzzle to arrive at an accurate diagnosis.

Diagnostic Evaluation of Sjogren's Syndrome

A diagnostic evaluation for patients with suspected Sjogren's syndrome usually includes the following:

- Patient medical history
- Physical examination
- Oral examination
- Ocular examination

- Laboratory studies
- Other studies

Patient History

A detailed patient history is crucial in the diagnostic "work-up" for Sjogren's syndrome. Information gathered by the doctor usually includes:

- History of symptoms - oral and ocular changes, fatigue, anxiety, joint or muscle pain
- Duration and pattern of symptoms
- Medications that the patient is presently taking that may cause similar symptoms
- History of other comorbid diseases

Physical Examination

The physical examination relating to the diagnosis of Sjogren's syndrome is very important because it may reveal certain important aspects of the disease, including:

- Salivary gland enlargement
- Regional lymph node swelling and tenderness
- Severely cracked lips
- Ulceration of the tongue
- Smooth tongue with atrophy of the papillae (taste buds)
- Halitosis - bad breath
- Pooling of saliva in the floor of the mouth
- Appearance of the eyes (e.g., red, watery)
- Excess production of mucus in lower part of eyes

Oral Examination

Studies that are performed to evaluate the extent and severity of oral symptoms in order to reach a diagnosis of Sjogren's syndrome include:

- *Sialometry* - This is a test which measures salivary flow rate. Collection devices are placed over the various salivary glands while saliva flow is stimulated with citric acid. It evaluates stimulated and unstimulated saliva flow rates for a set period of time. A flow rate of 0.5L or less in one minute for stimulated saliva, or a flow rate of 0.5L or less in five minutes for unstimulated saliva is indicative of *xerostomia* (reduction of salivary production). This test cannot, however, distinguish between the various possible causes of xerostomia.
- *Parotid sialography* - This is a radiographic evaluation of the salivary duct system to reveal any gross distortions of the parotid ductules such as a stone or a mass. An iodine-containing contrast material is introduced into the ductal system and the distribution pattern of the contrast dye through the salivary ducts is observed.

- *Salivary (parotid) gland scintigraphy* - This test is used to measure the timed uptake and excretion of a radioactive compound (*technetium*) by the major salivary glands and is a sensitive indicator of salivary gland function. It is also known as *radionuclide imaging*. In patients with Sjogren's syndrome, the uptake of the radioactive technetium compound is delayed and excretion into the oral cavity may not be noted at all.
- *Minor salivary gland biopsy* (also called lip gland biopsy) - A sample of the minor salivary glands of the lower lip is obtained and examined under a microscope to measure the extent of mononuclear cell infiltration. A *Focus Score* (the number of mononuclear cell infiltrates containing at least 50 inflammatory cells in a 4 mm2 glandular section) of one or higher, is considered to be consistent with Sjogren's syndrome. This highly specific test for the components of saliva in Sjogren's syndrome patients was in the past the "gold standard" technique used to diagnose Sjogren's syndrome (diagnostic criteria have since changed; see below). It may cause temporary soreness, but healing is rapid with no significant scarring.
- *Parotid gland biopsy* - performed in the presence of parotid gland swelling where lymphoma may be suspected.
- Dental examination - a careful dental examination by a dentist should be performed to evaluate the presence of rampant tooth decay (dental caries) which may be one of the first signs of dry mouth.

Eye Examination

Tests to evaluate the extent and severity of dry eye include:

- *Schirmer test* - This test is designed to evaluate the extent of dry eye by measuring the amount of tear production. In this test, a sterile filter paper strip is placed beneath the lower eyelid and the moistened area is measured after five minutes. Patients with Sjogren's syndrome usually produce less than 8 mm of tears (some of the literature cites five mm), while the normal response is 15 mm or more.
- *Slit-lamp examination* - This test is performed in conjunction with the Rose-Bengal dye test. Rose-Bengal dye is introduced into the conjunctival sac of the eye. The dye stains the corneal cells and can identify keratoconjunctivitis sicca (KCS) even when minimal ocular symptoms are present. After blinking twice, the slit-lamp examination evaluates the cornea for evidence of punctuate keratopathy (corneal irritation) and can detect destroyed conjunctival tissue which may be due to KCS.

Since keratoconjunctivitis sicca can be associated with other medical conditions, neither of these eye examinations alone is diagnostic for Sjogren's, but positive results of both tests combined confirms the diagnosis of Sjogren's syndrome.

Laboratory Studies

Laboratory studies that are performed to determine the presence of important markers of Sjogren's syndrome include:

- *Antinuclear Antibodies* (ANA) - Approximately 90% of patients with primary Sjogren's syndrome have elevated antinuclear antibodies (ANA) in their blood suggestive of an autoimmune disorder.
- *Rheumatoid Factor* (RF) - About 60% of patients with primary Sjogren's syndrome have elevated rheumatoid factor (RF) in their blood which is also consistent with an autoimmune disorder. It is important to note that detection of elevated levels of ANA or RF is not specifically diagnostic for Sjogren's syndrome since these substances may also be elevated in a broad range of other autoimmune, inflammatory, or infectious disorders.
- The presence of so-called *"Sjogren's antibodies"* (Ro/SS-A and La/SS-B) in the blood is more specific for Sjogren's syndrome; however, these antibodies are also detected in a significant number of patients with systemic lupus erythematosus (SLE).
- *Immunoglobulin* levels - Approximately 80% of patients with Sjogren's syndrome show signs of diffuse *hypergammaglobulinemia* (abnormally high levels of antibodies in the blood), specifically elevated levels of IgG, IgM, and IgA antibody subtypes.

Other Laboratory Studies

- Complete Blood Count (CBC) - Blood tests for Sjogren's syndrome may reveal several abnormalities including:

  - leucopenia - reduced number of white blood cells
  - thrombocytopenia - reduced number of platelets
  - anemia - reduced number of red blood cells

- Erythrocyte Sedimentation Rate (ESR) - elevated for the majority of Sjogren's syndrome patients

- Chest X-ray
- Other tests may be ordered by your doctor depending upon your specific symptoms

Upon diagnosis, the physician may see partial glandular destruction leading to dysfunction of remaining tissue. In addition, evidence of dry eye must be carefully evaluated as it is important to establish if the level of dry eye is compatible with the level of Sjogren's syndrome. Thus the doctor must make sure that the objective signs of dry eye are in agreement with the level of symptoms reported by the patient. In addition, while the lack of saliva may be a prominent symptom reported by the patient, it is not associated with any pain. If the patient complains of pain, other conditions causing dry mouth should be explored.

Controversy in the Diagnosis of Sjogren's Syndrome

The specific diagnostic criteria required for Sjogren's syndrome has been a source of controversy in the medical community in the past. The lack of a universally accepted classification system has contributed to the controversy and has made the clinical diagnosis of Sjogren's syndrome problematic. For example, different diagnostic criteria for patients with suspected Sjogren's syndrome have been used in the past by doctors in the United States, Europe, and Japan.

In 2002, a European-American consensus committee approved a set of six diagnostic criteria that is believed to be 95% accurate for the diagnosis of Sjogren's syndrome. The criteria were confirmed and published again in 2009 in the *American Family Physician* (vol.79(6):465-470) and include:

- Ocular symptoms
- Ocular signs
- Oral symptoms
- Salivary gland involvement
- Histopathology (microscopic examination of tissue)
- Laboratory results

Ocular Symptoms (at least one of the following symptoms must be present):
- Daily persistent troublesome dry eyes for at least three months
- Recurrent sensation of sand or gravel in the eyes
- Use of tear substitutes more than three times a day

Ocular Signs (at least one of the following signs must be present):
- Positive response for Schirmer eye test without anesthetic (5 ml or less of tears produced in 5 minutes)
- Ocular dye score (Rose-Bengal test or other) of 4 or higher

Oral Symptoms (at least one of the following symptoms must be present):
- Daily feeling of dry mouth for more than three months
- Recurrent or chronic swollen salivary glands as an adult

- Frequent drinking of liquid to help swallow dry food

Abnormal Salivary Gland Involvement (at least one of the following tests must be positive):
- Parotid gland scintigraphy
- Parotid sialography
- Sialometry response (unstimulated) of 1.5 mL or less in 15 minutes

Histopathology
- *Focus score* of 1 or higher (50 or more lymphocytes per 4 sq. mm of glandular tissue) in a minor salivary gland biopsy

Autoantibodies
- Presence of Ro(SS-A) and/or La (SS-B) antigens

For a definitive diagnosis of Sjogren's syndrome, at least one element in four of these six categories must be present and one of those positive elements must be either a positive histology response (focus score of more than 1) or the presence of SS-A/B autoantibodies. It is suggested that ANA be used to confirm the diagnosis rather than as an independent criterion, since up to 30% of healthy individuals may present with elevated ANA.

The European-American consensus group recommended that the following medical conditions be ruled out before a patient with dry eye and dry mouth can be positively diagnosed with Sjogren's syndrome:

- Hepatitis C
- HIV infection (the virus that causes AIDS)
- Lymphoma
- Prior head and neck radiation
- Sarcoidosis
- Graft-versus-host disease (in bone marrow transplant patients)
- Use of anticholinergic drugs

Diagnostic criteria notwithstanding, the European-American consensus group acknowledged that an experienced clinician who is an expert in the area of clinical observation and diagnosis of Sjogren's syndrome is crucial for reaching a correct diagnosis of this condition.

Differential Diagnosis of Sjogren's Syndrome

Sjogren's syndrome is often misdiagnosed when the symptoms are evaluated separately, and a complete diagnostic picture is not considered. For example, the fatigue and joint or muscle pain experienced by many patients with Sjogren's syndrome is often misdiagnosed as fibromyalgia or chronic fatigue syndrome. A variety of other conditions or medications can produce signs and symptoms that may overlap with Sjogren's syndrome and should be considered in the differential diagnosis. These include:

Dry Eye

Conditions which can cause dry eyes include:

- Inflammation (e.g., Stevens-Johnson syndrome, chronic conjunctivitis, blepharitis)
- Medications (e.g. anticholinergics)
- Neurologic conditions that may interfere with tear production
- Amyloidosis - a buildup of amyloid protein in body tissues and organs)
- Sarcoidosis (a rare inflammation of the lymph nodes and other tissue)
- Blink abnormality
- Eyelid scarring
- Trauma to the eye
- Tumors
- Environmental conditions
- Other medical conditions (e.g. autoimmune diseases)

Dry Mouth

Conditions other than Sjogren's syndrome that may cause dry mouth include:

- Viral infections
- Diabetes mellitus
- Amyloidosis
- Sarcoidosis
- Trauma
- Radiation therapy
- Parkinson's disease
- Dehydration
- Infection
- Anxiety

Medications that can cause dry mouth include:

- Antihypertensives (blood pressure medication)
- Parasympatholytic agents
- Psychotherapeutic agents

Parotid Gland Enlargement

In addition to Sjogren's syndrome, other underlying conditions that can cause parotid gland enlargement include:

- Viral infections (e.g., HIV, hepatitis C, mumps)
- Metabolic diseases (e.g., diabetes, chronic pancreatitis, liver cirrhosis)
- Endocrine disorders (e.g., acromegaly or gonadal hypofunction)

Differential diagnosis of Sjogren's syndrome is very important not only for diagnostic purposes but for treatment of systemic aspects of Sjogren's syndrome as well. This is particularly important when considering other autoimmune conditions such as scleroderma, systemic lupus erythematosus, or rheumatoid arthritis, since they can present with nonspecific symptoms that are similar to those of Sjogren's syndrome (e.g., low fever, joint pain, or Raynaud's phenomenon).

Diagnosis of Secondary Sjogren's Syndrome

The diagnosis of secondary Sjogren's syndrome requires the following:

- Presence of an underlying connective tissue disorder
- One sicca syndrome (dry eye or dry mouth)
- Two signs (objective measures) of dry mouth and dry eye

Treatment Options for Sjogren's Syndrome

Despite extensive past and ongoing research, there is still no known cure for Sjogren's syndrome. Treatment involves a multidisciplinary team that includes ophthalmologists, dentists, and rheumatologists. In addition to the professional team, it is very important for patients to educate themselves about their condition and learn how they can participate in their treatment and maintain treatment compliance.

Goals of Treatment for Sjogren's Syndrome

The goals of treatment for Sjogren's syndrome include:

- Controlling the symptoms
- Preventing or limiting organ involvement
- Improving quality of life

Treatment for Sjogren's syndrome varies from patient to patient depending upon the priority of symptoms that need to be addressed. It is important to always be vigilant regarding the development of any secondary infections. Patients with primary Sjogren's syndrome and cryoglobulinemia (presence of cryoglobulins in the blood) may require closer monitoring and management since some studies indicate a relationship between cryoglobulinemia and a higher risk for serious complications.

To read more in-depth information about current and prospective therapies for Sjogren's syndrome, please click on the following link:
http://www.ncbi.nlm.nih.gov/pubmed/17714766

In general, there are two types of treatments for Sjogren's syndrome:

- Local, palliative measures and medications that focus specifically on the sicca syndrome (dry mouth and dry eyes)
- Systemic treatments for severe sicca symptoms and wider systemic involvement. These medications, discussed in more detail below, include:
    - antinflammatory agents
    - immunosuppressive drugs
    - biological agents or immunomodifying drugs

Palliative Measures to Treat Sicca Symptoms

Dry Mouth Symptoms

Some of the therapies with which dry mouth and its symptoms are managed include:

- Saliva substitutes
- Saliva stimulants
- Interferon-alpha
- Rebamipide
- Meticulous observance of oral hygiene
- Lifestyle modifications

Saliva Substitutes

Research to develop products that mimic the unique properties and characteristics of saliva has been disappointing so far. There are, however, products available known as saliva substitutes that are designed to replicate the lubricating and wetting function of natural saliva. They are used mostly by patients with moderate to severe dry mouth, since they must be applied frequently, and patients with less severe symptoms find this very inconvenient. In addition, many find the taste of the saliva substitutes to be unappetizing.

Saliva substitutes are formulated either as rinses, sprays, lozenges, swabs, or gels. Most contain carboxymethylcellulose, mucin, or glycerine that help lubricate the oral mucosa. Examples of saliva substitutes include:

- Glandosane™
- Moi-Stir™
- Salivart™
- Oralbalance™ - a moisturizing gel reported to be longer-lasting than others, usually used at night

Individuals should speak to their health care provider or to their pharmacists regarding the benefits of each type of saliva substitute and to help evaluate which one would be most effective. Sometimes more than one may be tried before obtaining relief for dry mouth.

Saliva Stimulants

Hydration of the mouth is a mainstay of nonpharmaceutical measures for managing dry mouth. There are various methods used to stimulate saliva including:

- Frequent ingestion of sugar-free drinks
- Chewing sugar-free gum
- Sucking sugar-free lozenges
- Sucking *maltose* lozenges such as Natrol Dry Mouth™ that contains anhydrous crystalline maltose (ACM). ACM stimulates saliva production for patients who retain

residual functional glandular tissue. It has been shown to objectively increase secretions and improve subjective reports of oral symptoms in patients with Sjogren's syndrome. The lozenges can be taken three times a day.
- Muscarinic agents

Muscarinic Agents

If the patient finds these suggestions inadequate, there are medications that have been developed to treat sicca symptoms. Research actively continues to identify medications that effectively stimulate the production of saliva and tears to relieve symptoms of the sicca syndrome. Drugs known as *secretagogues* (general secretory stimulants) or *sialogogues* (salivary stimulants) are designed to stimulate the production of saliva in patients who have some residual salivary gland function.

The most commonly used sialogogues are *muscarinic agonists* that stimulate the M1 and M3 receptors on the salivary glands resulting in increased salivary secretion, and they have been found to be highly effective. Significant subjective and measurable objective improvement is associated with these drugs. Approximately 60% of patients notice improvements of dry mouth symptoms with secretory stimulant drugs. They are usually well tolerated and not associated with significant side effects.

Muscarinic agonists approved by the U.S. Food and Drug Administration (FDA) for the treatment of dry mouth associated with Sjogren's syndrome are *pilocarpine* and *cevimeline*.

Pilocarpine (Salagen™)

This drug was approved by the FDA for the treatment of dry mouth in 1998. Some patients also report relief from symptoms of dry eye when using this drug. Typically, salivary flow rate is reported to increase within 15 minutes of administering the drug and a peak flow rate is maintained for up to four hours. Pilocarpine is classified as a Pregnancy Category C drug, meaning that animal studies have shown an adverse effect on the fetus, but there are no adequate and well-controlled studies on pregnant women. Side effects are usually well tolerated and tend to decrease over time and may include:

- Sweating
- Flushed face
- Diarrhea
- Increased urinary frequency
- Gastrointestinal disturbances
- Hypotension
- Rhinitis (runny nose)

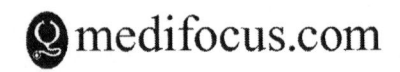

Pilocarpine is contraindicated in patients with Parkinson's disease.

Cevimeline (Evoxac™)

This is a newer muscarinic agonist agent that is more targeted for stimulating saliva production and has less of a systemic stimulatory effect than pilocarpine. It also increases secretion of sweat and tears. Cevimeline was approved by the FDA for the treatment of dry mouth in 2000. Results from a study regarding the efficacy and dosage of cevimeline indicated that patients taking 30 mg 3-4 times daily experienced statistically significant improvement of symptoms of dry mouth after six weeks of therapy and reported reduction of use of artificial saliva. Cevimeline reaches peak concentration in the blood after approximately one hour when taken without food. The duration of its effect is not clear. Cevimeline is also classified as Category C for pregnant women.

Adverse effects may include:

- Headache
- Sweating
- Abdominal pain
- Nausea (this is the most frequent side effect)

Typically patients who respond to muscarinic agonists are patients who exhibit:

- Less severe disease
- Shorter duration of sicca symptoms
- Less severe reduction of immunological markers (such as C3 or C4)
- Milder lymphocytic infiltration into the execretory glands

Muscarinic agonists are not recommended for patients with conditions that may be aggravated by muscarinic stimulation such as:

- Asthma
- Narrow-angle glaucoma
- Peptic ulcer disease
- Liver disease
- Acute iritis
- Severe cardiovascular disease
- Kidney stones
- Diarrhea

Interferon-Alpha

Oral interferon-alpha in the form of lozenges has been reported to significantly increase salivary stimulation and output. This oral formulation of interferon-alpha did not produce side effects typically associated with interferon given systemically (e.g., flu-like symptoms, fever, and malaise). Investigation of this drug for the treatment of dry mouth is ongoing.

Rebamipide

Rebamipide (Mucosta™) has been in clinical use in Japan and other Asian countries for almost 20 years for the treatment of gastritis (inflammation of the lining of the stomach) and gastric ulcers. Previous studies have shown that rebamipide exhibits anti-inflammatory properties and can also stimulate saliva production in an animal (rat) model of Sjogren's syndrome. Because of its anti-inflammatory and salivary production stimulation properties, rebamipide appears to be a promising candidate as an effective treatment for the treatment of dry mouth symptoms in patients with Sjogren's syndrome.

In a study published in 2009 in *Modern Rheumatology* (Volume 19; pp. 114-124), researchers from Japan reported the results of a double-blind, placebo-controlled trial of rebamipide for the treatment of dry mouth symptoms in 100 patients with Sjogren's syndrome who were randomly assigned to one of the following two groups:

- Rebamipide Group - 50 patients in this group received rebamipide (100 mg tablets) orally three times a day for eight weeks. Of these 50 patients, 37 had primary Sjogren's syndrome while 13 had been diagnosed with secondary Sjogren's syndrome.
- Placebo Group - 50 patients in this group received placebo tablets orally three times a day for eight weeks. The placebo tablets were indistinguishable in appearance and packaging from the rebamipide tablets. Thirty five patients in this group had primary Sjogren's and 15 had secondary Sjogren's syndrome.

After the start of the study, all of the participants were recalled weekly for the eight-week duration of the study and were evaluated using the following criteria:

- Overall improvement in dry mouth symptoms as reported by the patients (subjective evaluation)
- Changes in the volume of saliva secretion from before the start of the study and at weekly intervals for eight weeks
- Clinical examination of the oral cavity to determine improvement in the severity of dry mouth symptoms (objective evaluation)
- Laboratory tests (blood tests and urinalysis) to check for any abnormalities that may have developed due to treatment with either rebamipide or placebo tablets.

Based upon the data obtained during the eight-week course of this clinical trial, the Japanese researchers reported the following major findings:

- Overall improvement in dry mouth symptoms associated with Sjogren's syndrome was higher (although not statistically significant) in the rebamipide group as compared to the placebo group at all measurement time points over the eight-week course of the study.
- Dry mouth symptoms tended to show higher rates of improvement in the rebamipide section of the study in test subjects with *primary* Sjogren's syndrome as well as in subjects who were younger than 65 years in age.
- Although the rebamipide group showed a tendency toward increased salivary production with continuation of treatment as compared to the placebo group, the measured difference in salivary secretion among the two groups was not statistically significant.
- Further stratification of the data, however, revealed a statistically significant increase in salivary production favoring the rebamipide group among the subgroup of patients with *primary* Sjogren's syndrome. No increase in salivary production, however, was noted in the rebamipide group as compared to the placebo group among the subgroup of patients with *secondary* Sjogren's syndrome
- Laboratory studies of blood and urine in test subjects treated with rebamipide showed no abnormal findings from baseline. The most frequently reported side-effects during the eight-week course of the study were gastrointestinal disorders which were observed about equally in both the rebamipide and placebo groups.

In summary, this prospective, double-blind, placebo-controlled trial demonstrated the potential benefits of rebamipide for the treatment of dry mouth symptoms in patients with Sjogren's syndrome. A key observation noted in this study was the finding that treatment with rebamipide significantly improved both dry mouth symptoms as well as the volume of salivary production in patients with *primary*- but not *secondary*-Sjogren's syndrome. The authors of the study attributed this finding to the fact that almost 50% of the test subjects in the rebamipide section of the study were concomitantly receiving corticosteroid medications to treat the various connective tissue diseases (e.g., rheumatoid arthritis and systemic lupus erythematosus) that accompany *secondary* Sjogren's syndrome. Because corticosteroids are also potent anti-inflammatory medications that have previously been shown to have an improving effect on the symptoms of Sjogren's syndrome, the concomitant use of these medications by test subjects in this study with *secondary* Sjogren's syndrome may have "masked" the true overall benefits of rebamipide therapy.

The results of this study, involving a relatively small number of patients with Sjogren's syndrome, demonstrated that rebamipide appears to be a safe and potentially effective agent for the treatment of dry mouth symptoms in patients with *primary* Sjogren's syndrome. The authors noted, however, that additional studies are necessary to confirm the clinical efficacy of rebamipide before the drug can be brought into widespread clinical use.

Adherence to Good Oral Hygiene Practices

For patients with Sjogren's syndrome, developing good oral hygiene practices is an integral part of the overall strategy to prevent secondary complications of dry mouth such as dental caries (tooth decay), severe gum disease, and oral infections. Good oral hygiene practices include:

- Having regular dental checkups and cleanings by a dentist that can help prevent major dental problems. The cost of preventive dental care is considerably less than that associated with treating major dental problems.
- Brushing teeth twice a day with fluoride-based, low-abrasive toothpaste using a soft-bristled toothbrush; floss daily to keep teeth and mouth clean.
- Using products such as Dry Mouth Gum™, Toothpaste, or Mouth Wash made by Lacleade, Inc. have been reported to be beneficial for relief from dry mouth.
- Using sodium fluoride rinse daily and keep it in the mouth for at least one minute before expectorating. If using a fluoride gel, it should be applied with a toothbrush and kept in the mouth for two to three minutes, and then wait at least 30 minutes before eating or drinking
- Rinsing the mouth frequently with water - especially after meals - to keep it moist and clean.
- Avoiding snacks and candies that contain sugar. *Xylitol* is a naturally occurring sugar substitute that has been shown to reduce cavities when used in chewing gum.
- Checking the mouth routinely for signs of oral ulcers or infection such as red, white, or dark patches.
- Seeing a dentist promptly if any symptoms of oral infection are suspected, or if any other dental-related problems such as gingival (gum) inflammation develop.

Lifestyle Modifications

A variety of lifestyle modifications can help individuals with Sjogren's syndrome better control the symptoms of dry mouth and make them feel more comfortable as they go through normal daily activities. Some suggested modifications include:

- Chew gum or suck on hard candy (especially lemon) to stimulate the salivary glands.
- Be sure to choose sugar-free gum and candies to prevent tooth decay.
- Always carry a bottle of water and take frequent sips throughout the day to keep the mouth moist and comfortable, or suck on ice chips.
- Some individuals find that eating carrots or celery also stimulates saliva production.
- Use a lip balm to keep your lips moist and to treat dry, cracked lips. Lubricants such as Orajel or glycerin swabs placed under dentures helps to relieve dryness, soreness, or cracking of mucosal tissue. Cold air humidifiers at night may also be helpful.
- Avoid smoking because it dries out oral tissue and aggravates the symptoms of dry mouth.

- Avoid alcohol (including alcohol-based mouthwashes) because it can aggravate the symptoms of dry mouth.
- Avoid acidic fruit juices and carbonated beverages.
- Avoid hot, spicy foods since they may aggravate the burning sensation of the mouth that many Sjogren's patients experience.
- Avoid foods and/or medications sweetened with sucrose. Try to use sugar-free food products, whenever possible. Xylitol is a naturally occurring sugar substitute that has been shown to actually decrease cavities in the general population when used in chewing gum. It can also be purchased as a liquid or powder formulation for use in cooking.
- Avoid excessively hot or cold food.
- Avoid products containing sodium lauryl sulfate (found in soaps, shampoos, and toothpastes) since it may be associated with oral sores or ulcers.
- Do not wear dentures while sleeping. Rather soak them overnight to thoroughly clean them.
- Some patients have reported benefit from acupuncture and homeopathic remedies that stimulate salivary flow.
- Avoid medications that may worsen sicca symptoms by further depressing the functioning of the salivary glands, such as:

  - diuretics
  - antihypertensive medication (to control high blood pressure)
  - antidepressants
  - antihistamines

Treatment of Oral Candidiasis

Patients with Sjogren's syndrome are particularly susceptible to developing *oral candidiasis*, also called oral *thrush*, a fungal infection of the mouth characterized by whitish, velvety patches in the mouth and on the tongue. This condition can usually be treated with a topical antifungal agent such as nystatin (e.g., Mycostatin).

Dry Eye Symptoms

There are several products that are used and self-help tips that can be practiced in the management of dry eye syndrome in Sjogren's disease, including:

- Artificial tears
- Methylcellulose inserts
- Eye ointments
- Muscarinic agonist agents
- Immunomodulatory drugs

- Autologous serum eye drops
- Punctual occlusion surgery
- Life style modifications

Although topical nonsteroidal anti-inflammatory drugs may improve eye discomfort, they also reduce corneal sensitivity which elevates the risk for corneal damage. Patients using this class of drugs must be carefully monitored for any indication of side effects.

Artificial Tears
Artificial tears are most effective for relieving dry eye for patients with mild to moderate symptoms. Short acting preparations typically contain polymers such as carboxymethylcellulose or polyvinyl alcohol that increase the retention time of the tears on the eyes.

Some of these products contain various preservatives and/or salt which may cause eye irritation in some patients. Preservative-free artificial tears (e.g., Liquifilm™) are available over-the-counter and patients who use artificial tears on a daily basis find these to be less irritating to the eyes. A variety of artificial tear products are available on the market so if you are not sure which product to try, ask your eye doctor or pharmacist for recommendations.

Longer acting artificial tears preparations are formulated with either:

- Aqueous carbomer gels (e.g., Viscotears™, Geltears™)
- Paraffin (e.g., Lubri-Tears™, Lacri-Lube™)

Patients using the short-acting preparations (e.g., those based on carboxymethylcellulose) more than five or six times a day may consider switching to the longer-acting gels.

Methylcellulose Inserts
Hydroxypropyl methylcellulose inserts (Lacriserts) are small pellets that contain artificial tears and are inserted under the eyelid once daily to keep the surface of the eyes moist and wet. As a sustained-release formulation for artificial tears, the effect of the inserts can last anywhere from 6 to 12 hours making it suitable for nighttime use. Lacriserts are also effective for patients with dry eye whose symptoms cannot be controlled by frequent instillation of artificial tears.

Eye Ointments
Lubricating eye ointments (thicker than artificial tears) can provide relief of dry eye for several hours. One major drawback, however, is that they may cause blurry vision and for this reason many people prefer to use eye ointments just before going to sleep. Again, a variety of different products are available on the market and an eye doctor or pharmacist

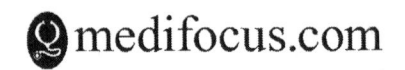

would be able to suggest the most effective ointment.

Muscarinic Agonists

Although muscarinic agonist (secretagogues) agents have been approved by the FDA only for xerostomia (dry mouth), some patients have found that they also have a beneficial effect on dry eyes. Dry eye symptoms may take longer to respond, with some patients experiencing relief after six to eight weeks of taking the drugs.

As noted in the treatment section for dry mouth, muscarinic agonists are contraindicated for patients with certain co-existing medical conditions, such as Parkinson's disease.

Immunosuppressant Drugs

Immunomosuppressant drugs include cyclosporine ophthalmic emulsion and corticosteroids.

Cyclosporine Ophthalmic Emulsion

Cyclosporine-A Ophthalmic Emulsion (Restasis™) is the first commercially available therapy for chronic dry eye disease that actually increases the production of natural tears. Phase III clinical trials of cyclosporine ophthalmic emulsions (0.05% and 0.1%) found significant improvement in tear production as measured by the Schirmer test. Restasis™ received approval in 2002 from the FDA for patients with moderate to severe dry eye disease due to deficiency in tear production. Oral cyclosporine did not prove effective for treatment of dry eye.

Adverse events associated with the use of Restasis™ include:

- Burning eye (most common side effect)
- Conjunctival hyperemia - engorgement of the conjunctival blood vessels
- Epiphora - watery eyes
- Stinging
- Foreign body sensation
- Visual disturbances - most commonly blurry vision

Tolerance for the side effects of Restasis™ usually develops with continued use.

Corticosteroids

- Topical corticosteroids - they target the inflammatory aspect of dry eye and have been shown to reduce corneal damage due to inflammation. Interestingly, objective test scores, such as Schirmers test, are not affected. Topical corticosteroids may also be effective as an acute treatment of inflammatory flare-ups of dry eye symptoms.

Side effects include:

- elevated intraocular pressure
- cataract formation when used for a period of a few weeks

- Loteprednol™, Rimexolone™ - oral corticosteroids that may be effective in improving signs and symptoms of dry eye.

Autologous Serum Eye Drops

Serum is the watery fluid found in blood that also moistens the surface of many membranes throughout the body. *Autologous* means that it is extracted from the patient's own blood. Serum is rich in proteins, vitamins, growth factors, and fibronectin, all of which are important for corneal and conjunctival health in the eye. It has also been shown that *albumin*, the major protein in serum, improved ocular surface damage. Autologous serum eye drops are non-allergenic and they have similar biochemical and biomechanical properties to natural tears. Several clinical trials have confirmed the advantage of autologous serum eye drops over conventional preservative-free artificial eye drops for keratoconjunctivitis sicca (dry eye) in patients with Sjogren's syndrome.

One of these trials was published in the *American Journal of Ophthalmology* in 2005 (vol.139(2):242-6) and compared signs and symptoms of severe dry eye in two groups of patients following the administration of preservative-free artificial tears or autologous serum eyedrops. Results indicated that signs (objective measures) and symptoms (subjective reporting) of dry eye improved significantly after two weeks in the group receiving autologous serum eyedrops.

Treatment with autologous serum eye drops continues to undergo investigation regarding the most effective formulation and doses. The formulation is also very costly since it must be based on the person's own blood.

To read more about autologous serum eye drops, please click on the following link:
http://www.ncbi.nlm.nih.gov/pubmed/18813071

Punctal Occlusion Surgery

For some patients whose symptoms of dry eye cannot be adequately controlled with conservative measures, *punctal occlusion surgery* may be a viable option. The goal of this surgery is to occlude (block) the tear ducts that drain tears from the eye. *Temporary punctal occlusion* involves surgically inserting collagen or silicone plugs into the tear ducts. A disadvantage of this treatment is that the plugs can fall out and get lost. *Permanent punctal occlusion* involves using a laser or electrocautery device to permanently seal-shut the tear ducts. This enables the tears to pool and, by doing so, provide much needed moisture to the eyes.

Lifestyle Modifications

There are a variety of modifications that patients with Sjogren's syndrome can make to help better control the symptoms of dry eye, including:

- Avoid smoking or areas where people smoke since smoke can aggravate the symptoms of dry eye.
- Use a humidifier in your home to maintain a comfortable relative humidity since dry air can aggravate ocular irritation from dry eye.
- Avoid air-conditioned places.
- When outdoors, wear dark or tinted glasses with side panels to protect your eyes from wind and bright sunlight in order to minimize tear loss.
- Avoid using contact lenses. Therapeutic contact lenses that are high in water content present a risk of dehydrating the conjunctiva which can increase the risk of infection since the protecting effect of tears is lacking. If using contact lenses, you may be advised to take prophylactic antibiotics and use lubricating agents frequently.
- Use eye ointment on the eyelids to minimize fluid loss from the mucous membranes.
- Some medications, such as tranquilizers and decongestants, increase the risk of dryness, and should be avoided if possible. Ask your doctor if some of the medications you may be taking may aggravate your symptoms of dry mouth and dry eye.
- Patients with Sjogren's syndrome who develop *blepharitis* (inflammation of the eyelid) as a complication of dry eyes may find relief by:

    - placing warm compresses on the eye
    - keeping the eyelid clean
    - applying a topical antibiotic as needed

- Avoid activities that can affect the tear film due to not blinking often enough, such as prolonged reading or looking at a computer screen.

- Try using goggles with moisture chambers in an environment that may aggravate symptoms.

Management of Dry Skin in Sjogren's Syndrome

Some patients with Sjogren's syndrome suffer from chronically dry skin and may benefit from the following suggestions:

- Apply moisturizing creams or lotions several times a day to keep your skin moist and

soft.
- Blot your skin dry after bathing or showering leaving a little moisture on your skin and then apply a moisturizing cream or lotion to help trap the moisture.
- Use aqueous creams and emollients rather than soap when bathing or showering.
- Avoid wearing tight-fitting clothing.
- Use a mild topical corticosteroid cream for mild itching of the skin.
- Avoid prolonged exposure to sunlight. If your skin is sensitive to sunlight, use a sunscreen to protect your skin.

Systemic Treatments for Severe Sicca Syndrome and Extraglandular Sjogren's Syndrome

With the exception of pilocarpine and cevimeline to treat dry mouth symptoms, there are no medications that have been approved by the U.S. Food and Drug Administration (FDA) for treatment of severe glandular or extraglandular symptoms associated with Sjogren's syndrome. Disease modifying antirheumatic drugs (DMARDs) such as those used for rheumatoid arthritis and systemic lupus erythematosus (SLE) have had limited success in the treatment of severe primary Sjogren's syndrome, though they may be effective on a limited basis in managing extraglandular manifestations. Medications to treat Sjogren's syndrome and the systemic manifestations are chosen on the basis of what seems to work for other patients and are modified on an as-needed basis.

In general, medications used for the treatment of severe Sjogren's syndrome and various systemic manifestations of Sjogren's syndrome include:

- Anti-inflammatory drugs, such as aspirin, Motrin or Advil. Some of these medications may be administered as a topical cream or suppository for patients who have difficulty swallowing pills.
- Immunosuppressive drugs

    - corticosteroids (e.g., prednisone) - Use is limited by their side effects, which include: osteoporosis, diabetes, mood changes, and cardiovascular changes. In addition, they accelerate the development of periodontal disease and oral candidiasis.
    - methotrexate (Trexall™)
    - azathioprine (Imuran™) - studies regarding the efficacy of this drug have so far been inconclusive.
    - cyclophosphamide (Cytoxan™) - an alkylating agent used to treat many types of cancer. In Sjogren's syndrome, it may be effective for potentially life threatening conditions but it is used with caution due to the high risk of lymphoma. To minimize this risk, some clinicians recommend pulse treatment

rather than daily administration.
- cyclosporine

- Disease Modifying Antirheumatic Drugs (DMARDs)

    - hydroxychloroquine (Plaquenil™) - regular eye checkups are recommended when taking this drug since an uncommon side effect is accumulation of this drug in the eye.
    - leflunomide (Arava™)

- Biological agents (immunomodifying drugs)

    - infliximab (Remicade™)
    - rituximab (Rituxan™)
    - interferon-alpha
    - etanercept (Enbrel™) - data regarding the efficacy of etanercept is not conclusive
    - eculizumab (Soliris™)

- Other medications:

    - thalidomide (Thalomid™)
    - dehydroepiandrosteron (DHEA)
    - octreotide (Sandostatin™)
    - antiviral agents
    - vitamin b12

Biological Agents

Biological agents target specific factors in the autoimmune response, such as B-cells and T-cells. Medications that result in B-cell depletion would be a major advance for the treatment of glandular and extraglandular symptoms in patients with Sjogren's syndrome since many are associated with excessive proliferation of B-cells. Anti-B-cell medications for Sjogren's syndrome have not been approved by the FDA at this time. They are used "off-label" (use of a medication for a condition for which it was not FDA-approved) for patients with severe cases of Sjogren's syndrome who are refractory to standard therapy of corticosteroids and other immunosuppressive agents, or patients with a life-threatening situation. The overall long-term risk of biological agents is unknown. Biological agents that are used to treat Sjogren's syndrome are *infliximab* and *rituximab*.

Infliximab (Remicade™) is a recombinant anti-tumor necrosis factor monoclonal antibody.

Data regarding the efficacy of infliximab have been inconclusive to date, with some small studies indicating significant improvement of symptoms. However, a 2004 multicenter, randomized, double-blind study clearly showed a lack of efficacy. It is not used as a first-line treatment but may be effective for some types of severe, refractory extraglandular features of Sjogren's syndrome.

Rituximab (Rituxan) is an anti-CD20 monoclonal antibody that appears to have an effect on B-cell hyperactivation which is closely associated with extraglandular symptoms and the development of B-cell lymphoma in Sjogren's syndrome. It was approved by the FDA in 2006 as a first line treatment of patients with diffuse large B-cell, CD20 positive non-Hodgkin's lymphoma in combination with other chemotherapy regimens. The FDA also approved rituximab for use in combination with methotrexate for reducing signs and symptoms in adult patients with moderately- to severely-active rheumatoid arthritis (an autoimmune disease) who have had an inadequate response to other therapies.

As noted above, rituximab has not been approved by the FDA for treatment of Sjogren's syndrome but several clinical trials with Sjogren's syndrome patients who were treated with rituximab have been conducted and have reported numerous benefits related to:

- Sicca syndrome
- Salivary gland production
- Extraglandular manifestations such as mixed cryoglobulinemia, refractory pulmonary disease, and peripheral neuropathy
- Fatigue
- Severe Sjogren's syndrome-related arthritis
- B-cell lymphoma - small studies have reported complete remission in some patients with MALT lymphoma.

Rituximab is typically administered with corticosteroids and not as a monotherapy. In 2006, the FDA issued a warning regarding fatal progressive multifocal leukoencephalopathy in patients with systemic lupus erythematosus (SLE) taking rituximab. This serious side effect has not been seen in patients with Sjogren's syndrome but clearly, patients on rituximab should be carefully monitored for the development of any neurological symptoms.

Additional potential adverse effects of rituximab include:

- Infusion reaction (up to 35% of cases)
- Neutropenia (abnormally low levels of neutrophils in the blood) occurs in up to 8% of patients
- Serum sickness (severe reaction due to the introduction of a foreign substance)

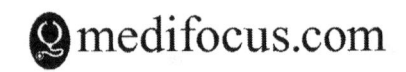

For further information about rituximab, please click on the following link:
http://www.ncbi.nlm.nih.gov/pubmed/19758218

Epratuzumab is another B-cell target therapy which was developed to treat non-Hodgkins lymphoma and has shown promising results for treatment with SLE. Belimumab, yet another monoclonal antibody against B-cells, has yielded promising results for patients with SLE and may potentially play a role in the future in treating Sjogren's syndrome. Small studies involving patients with Sjogren's syndrome are inconclusive but investigation is continuing on this promising medication.

Management of Musculoskeletal Symptoms

Muscle and joint pain associated with Sjogren's syndrome can usually be treated effectively with:

- Analgesics such as aspirin or non-steroidal anti-inflammatory drugs (e.g., Motrin™, Advil™) are the first-line of treatment for musculoskeletal symptoms
- Low-dose corticosteroid therapy (e.g., prednisolone) is usually reserved for patients suffering from:

    - severe joint pain or arthritis
    - cutaneous symptoms
    - severe oral and ocular sicca symptoms
    - myositis (inflammation of muscle tissue) and neuritis (nerve inflammation)

- Hydroxychloroquine (Plaquenil™) -Short term studies noted improvement in musculoskeletal symptoms (such as arthralgia, myalgia, malaise, or fatigue), as well as in some immune markers such as:

    - ANA - antinuclear antibody
    - rheumatic factor
    - erythrocyte sedimentation rate

Management of Fatigue

Patients with significant fatigue should also be evaluated and treated for other conditions such as:

- Depression
- Hypothyroidism
- Fibromyalgia
- Lymphoma

Exercise may be beneficial for some Sjogren's syndrome patients suffering from fatigue. Patients should consult their health care provider to determine what an appropriate level of exercise would be. A small study showed an improvement in fatigue after treatment with etanercept but there have not been any large-scale clinical trials which confirmed this finding. Hydroxychloroquine (Plaquenil™) may also be effective for treating fatigue in Sjogren's syndrome.

A small, double-blind, randomized controlled clinical trial was conducted in 2008 in which the authors studied the effect of rituximab on fatigue in primary Sjogren's syndrome. One group of patients received rituximab while the other group was given a placebo. Both groups received oral and intravenous steroids. There was a significant improvement in fatigue in the patients received rituximab compared to the placebo group. In addition, scores on tests for social functioning and mental health domains were significantly better at six months after treatment. To read more about this study, please click on the following link: http://www.ncbi.nlm.nih.gov/pubmed/18276741

Management of Vasculitis
Management of vasculitis may include:

- Corticosteroid creams
- Intravenous cyclophosphamide and high dose corticosteroids
- Plasma exchange (plasmapheresis) for severe complications of cryoglobulinemia vasculitis
- Intravenous immunoglobulins (IVIG)
- Rituximab

Raynaud's phenomenon may be treated with calcium-channel blockers or ACE (angiotensin-converting-enzyme) inhibitors. In addition, patients should try to avoid situations of physical or emotional stress.

Management of Pulmonary Symptoms
Severe pulmonary symptoms are rare in Sjogren's syndrome but, if they do develop, may be treated with corticosteroids. Pneumonia or bronchitis is typically treated with antibiotics. Some clinicians recommend immunization against pneumococcal infection. Use of a humidifier to keep the air moistened may also relieve some symptoms such as a dry, hacking cough.

Management of Renal Symptoms
Renal (kidney) involvement in patients with Sjogren's syndrome is typically subclinical. In severe cases, management may include:

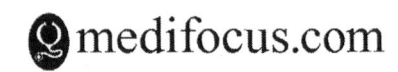

- Corticosteroid therapy
- Pulse intravenous cyclophosphamide combined with prednisolone for glomerulonephritis
- Oral potassium and sodium bicarbonate for acidosis
- Plasmapheresis (exchange of plasma)

Management of Gastrointestinal and Hepatobilliary Symptoms

- Gastroesophageal reflux can usually be controlled with medications such as antacids, histamine-2 (H-2) blockers, or proton-pump inhibitors.
- Sjogren's patients who develop mild hepatitis may require no specific treatment; however, liver function tests should be performed to monitor the course of the hepatitis. Patients with persistently elevated liver function tests may be treated with corticosteroids and azathioprine.
- Some patients with Sjogren's syndrome develop a condition called *primary biliary cirrhosis* that can lead to cirrhosis (hardening) of the liver. Treatments for primary biliary cirrhosis may include vitamin and calcium supplementation and other symptomatic treatments. In cases where liver damage is extensive, liver transplantation may be necessary.

Management of Neurological Symptoms

Peripheral and sensory neuropathies typically do not respond well to treatment but they often stabilize over time. Some patients with severe sensory neuropathy reported benefit from infliximab which may indicate that TNF-alpha drugs play a role in patients with other severe extraglandular involvement. Some patients with peripheral or cranial neuropathy report benefit from other medications such as:

- Corticosteroids
- Pulse intravenous cyclophosphamide combined with corticosteroids
- Azathioprine and methotrexate (if cyclophosphamide is not effective or not well tolerated)
- Low-dose antidepressants
- Anti-inflammatory agents
- Anticonvulsive agents (e.g., gabapentin)
- Plasmapheresis

Patients who fail to respond to more conservative measures should be thoroughly evaluated by a neurologist who can determine if there are other treatment options available.

Management of Gynecologic Symptoms

Vaginal lubricants can help make intercourse less painful. Vaginal estrogen creams increase capillary blood flow to the vaginal and vulvar area, thereby relieving vaginal dryness. Creams containing vitamin E or vitamin E oil are effective for lubricating the external vulvar surface and for relieving painful intercourse.

Examples of creams that may relieve vaginal dryness include:

- Replens™ (polycarbophil)
- Durex Sensilube™

Both of these creams are able to cling to the vaginal surface and rehydrate the surface cells and are effective for up to 72 hours. Cortisone creams should be avoided.

Management of Hematologic Symptoms

Hematologic symptoms associated with Sjogren's syndrome are managed with medications such as:

- Corticosteroids
- Immunosuppressants
- Azathioprine
- Cyclophosphamide
- Methotrexate
- Intravenous immunoglobulin (IVIG) combined with corticosteroids
- Plasmapheresis

Management of Lymphoproliferative Disorder

- Rituximab is a first-line therapy for B-cell lymphomas. Most lymphomas in Sjogren's patients are treated with the same protocols as lymphoma in the general population.
- Epratuzumab is under investigation for treatment of B-cell lymphoma.
- 2-chloro-2-deoxyadenosine is used for treatment of non-Hodgkin lymphoma (NHL) and is being investigated for treatment of NHL associated with Sjogren's syndrome.
- Interferon-alpha has been associated with decreased lymphocytic infiltration in some small studies.
- Hydroxychloroquine (for lymphadenopathy)

Summary of Treatment for Sjogren's Syndrome

Since there are no evidence-based therapeutic guidelines for management of Sjogren's syndrome (SS) related symptoms, a systematic review of treatments for primary Sjogren's syndrome was published in 2010 in the *Journal of the American Medical Association* (vol.304(4):pp.452-460). The review summarized the evidence regarding the efficacy of drugs used to treat the various aspects of SS. Results of 37 clinical trials that were reviewed indicated:

- Benefit for pilocarpine and cevilimene for sicca features
- Benefit for topical cyclosporine for moderate to severe dry eye
- Anti-tumor necrosis factor agents have not shown clinical efficacy
- Larger trials are needed to determine the efficacy of rituximab

In general, however, the review revealed low-level evidence for most of the drugs used for the treatment of SS and recommended the following:

- Dry eye
    - preservative-free tear substitutes and ocular ointments at night
    - topical cyclosporine (0.05% twice daily for moderate to severe dry eye
    - topical NSAIDs or glucocorticoids for patients with severe unresponsive dryness for as short a time as possible

- Dry mouth
    - saliva substitutes and sugar-free gum
    - avoidance of alcohol and smoking
    - thorough oral hygiene
    - pilocarpine and cevimeline, though their efficacy has never been compared in a clinical trial
    - N-acetylcysteine for patients who cannot tolerate those drugs

- General symptoms
    - no clear benefit noted for hydroxychloroquine (Plaquenil™) for muscle and joint pain or fatigue
    - off-label use of biologic agents for relief of general symptoms is not warranted

- Extraglandular symptoms
    - limited evidence for glucocorticoids and immunosuppressant drugs because studies were small and designed for treatment of sicca syndrome
    - rituximab showed improvement in vasculitis, neuropathy, glomerulonephritis, and arthritis
    - rituximab may be considered as a rescue drug for patients who are unresponsive to other treatments

- Life-threatening situations

- studies are limited but an expert review suggested methylprednisolone and cyclophosphamide pulses together with plasma exchanges for patients with rapidly progressing extraglandular symptoms or severe systemic vasculitis
- rituximab is used in life-threatening situations and for B-cell lymphoma

The authors note that B-cell targeted agents appear to be very promising for systemic relief of SS based on small studies. For in-depth information about treatment for SS, please click on the following link: http://www.ncbi.nom.nih.gov/pubmed/20664046.

Prognosis in Sjogren's Syndrome

Sjogren's syndrome is typically a benign process but has a significant impact on quality of life. Most dry mouth/eyes symptoms and musculoskeletal symptoms such as arthralgia and fatigue can be managed effectively with muscarinic agonists, corticosteroids, and several self-help techniques. Systemic therapy, including traditional antirheumatic drugs to alter the course of the disease and halt the decline of glandular function has not been effective. Regardless of treatment, though, salivary flow is lost over time and many patients will experience at least one episode of inflammatory arthritis in the course of the disease.

There is a subset of patients who develop severe sicca symptoms and extraglandular involvement. These patients require continued monitoring and aggressive treatment that may consist of corticosteroids, immunosuppressive agents, biological agents, and/or plasmapheresis. Aggressive therapy and monitoring is particularly important for patients whose symptoms and blood values place them at high risk for the development of lymphoma. Approximately 60% of patients exhibit antibodies against Ro/SS-A and La/SS-B. The presence of these antibodies is associated with:

- Early disease onset
- Longer disease duration
- Parotid gland enlargement
- Increased frequency of extraglandular involvement
- Greater infiltration of lymphocytes into the glands

Although patients with primary Sjogren's syndrome do not have a higher overall mortality rate as compared to the general population, they are at higher risk of dying from a lymphoproliferative condition such as lymphoma, which develops in approximately 5% of patients with primary Sjogren's syndrome. The most common types of lymphoma associated with Sjogren's disease are low-grade, marginal zone B-cell lymphoma and MALT, and are typically located in the parotid gland. Lymphoma is usually treated with rituximab and other standard chemotherapy treatment protocols. While there is no definitive evidence to support screening patients with Sjogren's syndrome for lymphoproliferative diseases, there are certain features which raise the index of suspicion for development of these diseases, including:

- Enlarged parotid glands
- Regional or general lymphadenopathy
- Hepatosplenomegaly (enlarged liver and spleen)
- Vasculitis
- Hypergammaglobulinemia (elevated gammaglobulin)
- Pulmonary infiltrates (airspaces in the lung fill with fluid and/or inflammatory cells)

In general, an adverse outcome for Sjogren's syndrome is associated with four factors present at diagnosis which require intensive monitoring, namely:

- Vasculitis
- Grades III-IV parotid scintigraphy (severe involvement)
- Hypocomplementemia (low C3/C4 levels in the blood)
- Cryoglobulinemia (low levels of cryoglobulins in the blood)

For further information about prognosis in Sjogren's syndrome, please click on the following link: http://www.ncbi.nlm.nih.gov/pubmed/17569749

Quality of Life Issues and Psychosocial Considerations in Sjogren's Syndrome

The impact of Sjogren's syndrome on quality of life is quite significant due to the multitude of functions that are affected, particularly dry mouth and dry eyes. Sjogren's syndrome takes a toll on the physical, psychological, economic, and social aspects of daily life of Sjogren's patients, and by extension, on their families and friends. For example, because Sjogren's patients suffering from dry eye may react to physical environments that aggravate their condition (e.g. air-conditioned places), they may refrain from going out with friends. A patient suffering from dry mouth may withdraw from family and friends due to the embarrassment of difficulties such as not speaking clearly or experiencing bad breath. In addition, the Sjogren's patient's self-perception may undergo changes that can lead to or exacerbate depression or anxiety. It is important for the patient with Sjogren's syndrome to address these and any other issues that are distressing to them with a team of health professionals.

Dry Mouth

The effects of dry mouth that can impact a patient's quality of life are numerous and include:

- Dietary habits
- Nutritional status due to difficulties chewing and swallowing
- Speech articulation
- Susceptibility to cavities
- Periodontal disease
- Oral/fungal infection
- Weakened jaw bone
- Reduced tolerance for dental prosthetics, (e.g., implants, bridges)

Dry Eyes

The effects of dry eye that can impact a patient's quality of life are also numerous and include:

- Dry, itchy eyes
- Corneal abrasion
- Irritation of the eyes
- Reduced self-image because of need to protect eyes

- Reduced employment opportunities due to environmental issues to protect the eyes

Lifestyle Modifications

Lifestyle modifications that may be helpful to overall comfort of the patient with Sjogren's syndrome and may improve the quality of life include:

- Avoid or minimize exposure to:

  - smoke
  - low humidity
  - forced hot air heating systems
  - excessive air conditioning

- If you smoke, STOP because smoking exacerbates the symptoms of Sjogren's syndrome.

- Use humidifiers to increase the comfort of your home or office environment. Remember, it is very important to clean the humidifier daily to prevent accumulation of germs.
- Add leafy plants to your environment since they help to promote moisture in the air.
- Increase fluid intake by frequently drinking fluids or by sucking on ice chips.
- Keep sugar-free gum close by and chew often.
- Suck on highly flavored lemon lozenges that helps promote stimulation of saliva.
- Keep lip salve available to prevent and treat dry cracked lips.
- Use glasses with side panels or goggles when you go outside to block the wind from drying out your eyes.
- Use aqueous creams and emollients rather than soap when washing.
- Following a bath or shower, blot the skin dry leaving some moisture on your skin and immediately apply a moisturizing cream.
- Wear loose clothing to alleviate suffering discomfort from skin-conditions.
- Schedule dental visits 2-3 times a year for teeth cleaning and evaluation.
- Rinse your mouth with water several times a day. Avoid alcohol-based mouthwashes which may add to the dryness of the mouth.
- After each meal, brush your teeth gently but thoroughly.
- Minimize sugary foods. If you do eat or drink a sugary product, brush your teeth and rinse out your mouth immediately afterwards.
- Floss regularly and inspect your mouth daily for any sores, redness, or bleeding. See a dentist if you notice any changes in your mouth.

Psychosocial Considerations

Participation with the healthcare team in order to maximize the extent of relief from various symptoms is very important. Cooperative efforts can be helpful regarding:

- Stress reduction
- Comfort management
- Pain management
- Acquisition of habits that reduce discomfort
- Preventing secondary complications, such as infections
- Treatment for depression or anxiety
- Adhering to scheduled visits with healthcare providers is important in order to:

    - monitor your clinical status
    - monitor laboratory tests
    - recognize and commence early treatment for any new complications which may develop

Women with Sjogren's syndrome often report that the lack of a definitive diagnosis is extremely frustrating and that their health care providers often do not take their symptoms seriously. Some report being told that they are neurotic or depressed. Many women report suffering for several years without a diagnosis. Part of the reason for this delay in diagnosis is that Sjogren's syndrome often appears around the age of menopause so that symptoms of Sjogren's syndrome may overlap with naturally occurring conditions such as increasing vaginal dryness. Vaginal dryness impacts quality of life significantly for some women as intercourse may be painful and there is a general discomfort from continued dryness. Sexual life is completely interrupted and the frustration is magnified when there is no help or support from health care providers.

It is essential for women to be educated about the symptoms of Sjogren's syndrome that may affect their daily lives, and to contact support groups, organizations, or professionals who may be able to provide advice, guidance, and appropriate treatment.

One of the major symptoms that many patients with Sjogren's syndrome find very debilitating is fatigue, which is described as an intense feeling of physical and mental exhaustion that can lead to:

- Emotional stress
- Depression
- Increased irritability and intolerance
- General lethargy

Related to fatigue is the common occurrence of fibromyalgia, which is reported by many Sjogren's syndrome patients. In addition to the medications that may be prescribed to control or minimize the pain of this condition, patients may benefit from trying various methods of coping with fibromyalgia, including:

- Regular exercise regimens that should be determined in cooperation with a health care provider
- Fast walking
- Physical therapy that may incorporate various modalities of treatment, including:
  - passive stretching exercises
  - massage treatment
  - application of heat compresses
  - lidocaine injections at pain trigger points

Patients with Sjogren's syndrome report that family and friends may not understand the extent of the impact of symptoms on their quality of life, which may in itself add to feelings of anxiety and depression. In addition, any major changes in the daily routine of a patient with Sjogren's syndrome may exacerbate physical and psychological stress. Patients who experience fatigue as one of their symptoms may benefit from modifying their behavior to maximize their energy levels. Modifications may include:

- Pacing daily activities or particular activities to preserve strength
- Modified exercise regimen
- Mental stimulation
- Relaxation exercises as needed during the day

When away from home (e.g., trips, vacations, office), it is important for patients with Sjogren's syndrome to remember to take along with them all of their sprays, gels, medications, and other items that aid in control of their symptoms.

New Developments in Sjogren's Syndrome

Researchers are continuing to investigate Sjogren's syndrome in hopes of gaining a deeper understanding about the pathophysiology of the disorder and using this information to develop novel approaches for improved treatments. Some of the current areas of research interest in Sjogren's syndrome include:

Therapies for Dry Mouth under Investigation for Sjogren's Syndrome

- Evaluation of a mouth rinse solution containing *casein derivative calcium phosphate* (CD-CP) to help prevent tooth decay in patients with dry mouth.
- Evaluation of *trithio-p-methoxyphenylpropene* (Sialor™) for stimulating salivary secretion in patients with dry mouth.
- Transplantation of submandibular salivary glands is in early stages of research as a potential treatment for xerostomia.
- A clinical trial investigating the drug *mizoribine* for treatment of sicca syndrome yielded promising results in patients' assessment of improvement. To read more about this treatment, please click on the following link: http://www.ncbi.nlm.nih.gov/pubmed/18506160
- There is an ongoing effort to produce saliva substitutes based on new thickening agents such as *linseed polysaccharide* or *xanthan gum polysaccharide* to achieve longer adherence on mucosal surfaces.
- Researchers are studying a treatment involving irrigation of the parotid gland with prednisolone.
- Efforts are underway to reformulate pilocarpine as a slow-release medication that will deliver medication at a slow, steady rate over a longer period of time than the present form.
- Researchers in Germany tested a device consisting of stimulating electrodes, an electronic circuit, and a power source for relief of dry mouth. Details of this study can be seen at http://www.ncbi.nom.nih.gov/pubmed/20882668. The two-staged study yielded the following results:

  - At the end of stage I (one month), the device was superior to a sham deice in providing relief to dry mouth severity, frequency, quality of life impairment, and swallowing difficulty.
  - At the end of stage II (three months) statistically significant improvements were verified for dry mouth severity, frequency, oral discomfort, speech difficulty, sleeping difficulty, and increased resting salivary output.

- Here is a link to an interesting study investigating the effect of homeopathic medicine on salivary flow rates: http://www.ncbi.nlm.nih.gov/pubmed/16060203

Dry Eye Therapies under Investigation for Sjogren's Syndrome

- Researchers at the Massachusetts Eye and Ear Infirmary in Boston investigated the efficacy of multiple daily dosing of topical cyclosporine 0.05% for patients with severe dry eye disease who did not respond to the usual twice-a-day regimen. Twenty-two patients were given topical cyclosporine 0.05% either three or four times a day for a two-month course of treatment. Overall dry eye symptoms improved in 15 patients (68%) and global physician assessment of dry eye status improved in 16 patients (72%). Three patients (13%) reported new symptoms of burning or irritation. The authors conclude that patients with severe dry eye symptoms that do not respond to a twice-daily regimen may require more frequent dosing of topical cyclosporine. To read more about this study, please click on the following link: http://www.ncbi.nlm.nih.gov/pubmed/19770713
- Cevimeline (Evoxac), a drug that has already been approved by the U.S. Food and Drug Administration (FDA) for the treatment of dry mouth, is also being evaluated as a potentially safe and effective treatment for dry eye.
- Topical therapy with cyclosporin A is being evaluated for the treatment of dry eye.
- Novel topical agents that are designed to enhance the transport of water across the conjunctiva by stimulating specific receptors in the eye known as purinogenic ocular surface receptors are being developed for the treatment of dry eye.
- Eye-drops formulated with *hyaluronate* show promise for the treatment of severe dry eye in Sjogren's patients.
- Novel secretogogues that target secretion of *mucins* which form the inner layer of the tear film and are responsible for lubrication and protection including:

    - INS365 (*diquafosol tetrasodium*) - improved test scores of Schirmer test and corneal/conjunctival staining
    - 15S-HETE
    - *ecabet sodium* - an anti-ulcer agent that has shown promise for treatment of dry eye
    - *gefarnate* - used in the treatment of gastric ulcers and has shown potential for treatment of dry eye

- Gene transfer of therapeutic agents (such as immunomodifying agents) into the affected gland has successfully been studied in animals. Researchers are investigating the potential of carrying out this model for treatment in humans.

Systemic Treatments under Investigation for Sjogren's Syndrome

- Researchers are investigating treatments not only for the dry eye and dry mouth symptoms but also to modify the progression of the disease. New approaches include interference with inflammation processes and chemical receptors as well as strategies to preserve and restore functional exocrine tissue. To read more about emerging treatment strategies and potential therapeutic targets in primary Sjogren's syndrome, please click on the following link: http://www.ncbi.nlm.nih.gov/pubmed/19906008

- To assess the effect of rituximab therapy on parotid tissue in Sjogren's disease, five patients underwent a parotid biopsy before starting a regimen of rituximab and subsequently underwent an addition parotid biopsy after 12 weeks of rituximab infusions. The authors concluded that the histopathologic evidence of reduced glandular inflammation seen in this small subset of Sjogren's patients may indicate the potential for glandular restoration with rituximab. To read more about this study, please click on the following link: http://www.ncbi.nlm.nih.gov/pubmed/19877054. Results of the study showed that following treatment:

    - four of the five patients showed an increased salivary flow rate and a normalization of salivary sodium concentration
    - lymphocytic infiltrate of the parotid gland was reduced in all five patients
    - in three patients, the amount and extent of a particular type of lesion was reduced, and in two patients, it was completely absent
    - the proliferation of cluster-like tissue that forms in response to inflammation was reduced in all patients

- Investigators studied the relationship between periodontal disease and Sjogren's syndrome. They found that there are several alterations to the capillaries that affect microcirculation of the gingiva in the mouths of patients with Sjogren's syndrome. More about this study can be seen at the following link: http://www.ncbi.nom.nih.gov/pubmed/19729367

- Results of a clinical trial investigating the treatment of autoimmune-related interstitial lung disease with *mycophenolate mofetil* (MMF) instead of cyclophosphamide (CYC) were published in 2009 in the *American Journal of Medical Science*. Cyclophosphamide is associated with significant toxicity and poor outcome. Ten patients received MMF while five patients received CYC infusion. Results were encouraging regarding MMF-treated patients who showed improvement

in alveolitis (diffuse interstitial lung disease), symptoms related to coughing, dyspnea, and chest discomfort, and perceived quality of life and activity levels. In addition, average doses of prednisone were reduced significantly without worsening of the patient's condition. To read more about this study, please click on the following link: http://www.ncbi.nlm.nih.gov/pubmed/19295413
- Research regarding development of biologic agents which target B-cells and T-cells in Sjogren's syndrome is very robust. NOTE: Efalizumab (Raptiva) is a medication that is used for the treatment of a condition called *psoriasis* - a chronic skin disease characterized by dry red patches covered with scales. In April 2009, this drug was withdrawn from the U.S. market due to the potential risk of patients developing *progressive multifocal leukoencephalopathy* - a usually fatal condition that is characterized by progressive brain damage due to inflammation of the white matter of the brain. Efalizumab (Raptiva) is no longer available in the U.S. as of June 8, 2009.

To read the summary of an article about B-cell depletion therapies that appeared in August of 2009 in *Autoimmunity Reviews*, please click on the following link: http://www.ncbi.nlm.nih.gov/pubmed/19671451

- Other medications being investigated for treatment of extraglandular involvement in Sjogren's syndrome include:

    - infliximab (Remicade)
    - etanercept (Enbrel)
    - thalidomide (Thalomid)
    - leflunomide (Arava)
    - 2-chlorodeoxyadenosine (Cladribine)
    - octreotide (Sandostatin)
    - azathioprine (Imuran)

For information regarding clinical trials being conducted for Sjogren's syndrome, please click on the following links: http://www.clincialtrials.gov or http://www.centerwatch.com

Questions to Ask Your Health Care Provider about Sjogren's Syndrome

- How can you be sure that my symptoms of dry mouth and/or dry eye are due to Sjogren's syndrome and not some other disorder?
- What types of diagnostic tests will I need to undergo in order to confirm the diagnosis?
- What types of treatments do you recommend for dry mouth?
- What types of treatments do you recommend for dry eye?
- What treatments will I need to undergo if I have Sjogren's syndrome with systemic involvement?
- Which types of physicians or other health care professionals should I have on my treatment team?
- Can you recommend any health care providers specializing in treating patients with Sjogren's syndrome?
- How should I expect my symptoms to progress over time?
- Are there any lifestyle modifications that may better control my symptoms?
- How often should I schedule follow-up visits for reevaluation?
- Should I be followed by each specialist separately or can one health care provider manage my condition?
- Are there any clinical trials focusing on new treatments for Sjogren's syndrome?

NOTES

Use this page for taking notes as you review your Guidebook

3 - Guide to the Medical Literature

Introduction

This section of your *MediFocus Guidebook* is a comprehensive bibliography of important recent medical literature published about the condition from authoritative, trustworthy medical journals. This is the same information that is used by physicians and researchers to keep up with the latest advances in clinical medicine and biomedical research. A broad spectrum of articles is included in each *MediFocus Guidebook* to provide information about standard treatments, treatment options, new developments, and advances in research.

To facilitate your review and analysis of this information, the articles in this *MediFocus Guidebook* are grouped in the following categories:

- Review Articles - 43 Articles
- General Interest Articles - 86 Articles
- Drug Therapy Articles - 9 Articles
- Clinical Trials Articles - 19 Articles

The following information is provided for each of the articles referenced in this section of your *MediFocus Guidebook*:

- Title of the article
- Name of the authors
- Institution where the study was done
- Journal reference (Volume, page numbers, year of publication)
- Link to Abstract (brief summary of the actual article)

Linking to Abstracts: Most of the medical journal articles referenced in this section of your *MediFocus Guidebook* include an abstract (brief summary of the actual article) that can be accessed online via the National Library of Medicine's PubMed® database. You can easily access the individual article abstracts online by entering the individual URL address for a particular article into your web browser, or by going to the following special URL:

http://www.medifocus.com/links/RH011/0112

Recent Literature: What Your Doctor Reads

Database: PubMed <January 2008 to January 2012>

Review Articles

1.

Treatment of Sjogren's syndrome-associated dry eye an evidence-based review.

Authors:	Akpek EK; Lindsley KB; Adyanthaya RS; Swamy R; Baer AN; McDonnell PJ
Institution:	The Wilmer Eye Institute, The Johns Hopkins University School of Medicine, Baltimore, MD, USA. esakpek@jhmi.edu
Journal:	Ophthalmology. 2011 Jul;118(7):1242-52. Epub 2011 Apr 3.
Abstract Link:	http://www.medifocus.com/abstracts.php?gid=RH011&ID=21459453

2.

The meaning of anti-Ro and anti-La antibodies in primary Sjogren's syndrome.

Authors:	Hernandez-Molina G; Leal-Alegre G; Michel-Peregrina M
Institution:	Immunology and Rheumatology Department, Instituto Nacional de Ciencias Medicas y Nutricion SZ, Vasco de Quiroga 15. Colonia Seccion XVI, CP 14000, Mexico City, Mexico. gabyhm@yahoo.com
Journal:	Autoimmun Rev. 2011 Jan;10(3):123-5. Epub 2010 Sep 15.
Abstract Link:	http://www.medifocus.com/abstracts.php?gid=RH011&ID=20833272

Go to http://www.medifocus.com/links/RH011/0112 for direct online access to the above Abstract Links.

3.

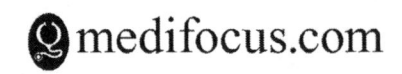

Dermatologic manifestations of Sjogren syndrome.

Authors:	Kittridge A; Routhouska SB; Korman NJ
Institution:	West Penn Allegheny Health System, Department of Medicine, Pittsburg, PA, USA.
Journal:	J Cutan Med Surg. 2011 Jan-Feb;15(1):8-14.
Abstract Link:	http://www.medifocus.com/abstracts.php?gid=RH011&ID=21291650

4.

A current perspective on Sjogren's syndrome.

Authors:	Nazmul-Hossain AN; Morarasu GM; Schmidt SK; Walker AJ; Myers SL; Rhodus NL
Institution:	Dental Research Institute, University of California, Los Angeles, USA.
Journal:	J Calif Dent Assoc. 2011 Sep;39(9):631-7.
Abstract Link:	http://www.medifocus.com/abstracts.php?gid=RH011&ID=22034797

5.

Biological therapies in primary Sjogren's syndrome.

Authors:	Ng WF; Bowman SJ
Institution:	University of Newcastle, Institute of Cellular Medicine, Musculoskeletal Research Group, Newcastle upon Tyne, NE2 4HH, UK. wan-fai.ng@ncl.ac.uk
Journal:	Expert Opin Biol Ther. 2011 Jul;11(7):921-36. Epub 2011 Apr 4.
Abstract Link:	http://www.medifocus.com/abstracts.php?gid=RH011&ID=21457124

Go to http://www.medifocus.com/links/RH011/0112 for direct online access to the above Abstract Links.

6.

Peripheral nervous system manifestations of Sjogren syndrome: clinical patterns, diagnostic paradigms, etiopathogenesis, and therapeutic strategies.

Author:	Birnbaum J
Institution:	Department of Neurology, The Johns Hopkins Jerome Greene Sjogren's Center, Baltimore, MD, USA. jbirnba2@jhmi.edu
Journal:	Neurologist. 2010 Sep;16(5):287-97.
Abstract Link:	http://www.medifocus.com/abstracts.php?gid=RH011&ID=20827117

7.

Primary Sjogren's syndrome activity and damage indices comparison.

Authors:	Campar A; Isenberg DA
Institution:	Santo Antonio Hospital - Centro Hospitalar do Porto, Porto, Portugal.
Journal:	Eur J Clin Invest. 2010 Jul;40(7):636-44. Epub 2010 May 17.
Abstract Link:	http://www.medifocus.com/abstracts.php?gid=RH011&ID=20482595

8.

Neurological manifestations of primary Sjogren's syndrome.

Authors:	Chai J; Logigian EL
Institution:	Department of Neurology, National NeuroScience Institute, Singapore.
Journal:	Curr Opin Neurol. 2010 Oct;23(5):509-13.
Abstract Link:	http://www.medifocus.com/abstracts.php?gid=RH011&ID=20689426

9.

Stem cells in the spleen: therapeutic potential for Sjogren's syndrome, type I diabetes, and other disorders.

Authors:	Faustman DL; Davis M
Institution:	Massachusetts General Hospital, Harvard Medical School, Charlestown, MA 02129, USA. faustman@helix.mgh.harvard.edu
Journal:	Int J Biochem Cell Biol. 2010 Oct;42(10):1576-9. Epub 2010 Jun 18.
Abstract Link:	http://www.medifocus.com/abstracts.php?gid=RH011&ID=20601088

Go to http://www.medifocus.com/links/RH011/0112 for direct online access to the above Abstract Links.

10.

Pulmonary involvement in Sjogren syndrome.

Authors:	Kokosi M; Riemer EC; Highland KB
Institution:	3rd Pulmonary Department, Sismanoglio General Hospital, Athens, Greece.
Journal:	Clin Chest Med. 2010 Sep;31(3):489-500.
Abstract Link:	http://www.medifocus.com/abstracts.php?gid=RH011&ID=20692541

11.

Pathogenesis of Sjogren's syndrome and therapeutic consequences.

Authors:	Mariette X; Gottenberg JE
Institution:	Hopital Bicetre, Assistance Publique-Hopitaux de Paris, Universite Paris-Sud 11, Institut Pour la Sante et la Recherche Medicale U1012, Le Kremlin Bicetre, France. xavier.mariette@bct.aphp.fr
Journal:	Curr Opin Rheumatol. 2010 Sep;22(5):471-7.
Abstract Link:	http://www.medifocus.com/abstracts.php?gid=RH011&ID=20671520

12.

Sjogren syndrome: more than dry eyes.

Authors:	Pullen RL Jr; Hall DA
Institution:	Amarillo College in Amarillo, Texas, USA.
Journal:	Nursing. 2010 Aug;40(8):36-41.
Abstract Link:	**ABSTRACT NOT AVAILABLE**

13.

Pulmonary amyloidosis in Sjogren's syndrome: a case report and systematic review of the literature.

Authors:	Rajagopala S; Singh N; Gupta K; Gupta D
Institution:	Department of Pulmonary Medicine, Postgraduate Institute of Medical Education and Research (PGIMER), Chandigarh, India. visitsrinivasan@gmail.com
Journal:	Respirology. 2010 Jul;15(5):860-6. Epub 2010 Jun 4.
Abstract Link:	http://www.medifocus.com/abstracts.php?gid=RH011&ID=20546191

Go to http://www.medifocus.com/links/RH011/0112 for direct online access to the above Abstract Links.

14.

Treatment of primary Sjogren syndrome: a systematic review.

Authors:	Ramos-Casals M; Tzioufas AG; Stone JH; Siso A; Bosch X
Institution:	Sjogren Syndrome Research Group (AGAUR), Josep Font Laboratory of Autoimmune Diseases, IDIBAPS, Department of Autoimmune Diseases, Hospital Clinic, C/Villarroel, 170, 08036 Barcelona, Spain. mramos@clinic.ub.es
Journal:	JAMA. 2010 Jul 28;304(4):452-60.
Abstract Link:	http://www.medifocus.com/abstracts.php?gid=RH011&ID=20664046

15.

Use of methotrexate in patients with systemic lupus erythematosus and primary Sjogren's syndrome.

Authors:	Winzer M; Aringer M
Institution:	Division of Rheumatology, Department of Medicine III, University Center Carl Gustav Carus, Technical University of Dresden, Dresden, Germany.
Journal:	Clin Exp Rheumatol. 2010 Sep-Oct;28(5 Suppl 61):S156-9. Epub 2010 Oct 28.
Abstract Link:	http://www.medifocus.com/abstracts.php?gid=RH011&ID=21044451

16.

Ocular surface injuries in autoimmune dry eye. The severity of microscopical disturbances goes parallel with the severity of symptoms of dryness.

Authors:	Cejkova J; Ardan T; Cejka C; Malec J; Jirsova K; Filipec M; Ruzickova E; Dotrelova D; Brunova B
Institution:	Department of Eye Histochemistry and Pharmacology, Institute of Experimental Medicine, Academy of Sciences of the Czech Republic, Prague, Czech Republic. cejkova@biomed.cas.cz
Journal:	Histol Histopathol. 2009 Oct;24(10):1357-65.
Abstract Link:	http://www.medifocus.com/abstracts.php?gid=RH011&ID=19688700

Go to http://www.medifocus.com/links/RH011/0112 for direct online access to the above Abstract Links.

17.

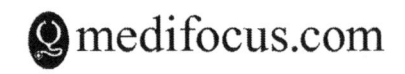

Emerging new pathways of pathogenesis and targets for treatment in systemic lupus erythematosus and Sjogren's syndrome.

Author:	Perl A
Journal:	Curr Opin Rheumatol. 2009 Sep;21(5):443-7.
Abstract Link:	http://www.medifocus.com/abstracts.php?gid=RH011&ID=19584730

18.

Patient-reported outcomes including fatigue in primary Sjogren's syndrome.

Author:	Bowman SJ
Institution:	Rheumatology Department, University Hospital Birmingham (Selly Oak), Birmingham B296JD, UK. simon.bowman@uhb.nhs.uk
Journal:	Rheum Dis Clin North Am. 2008 Nov;34(4):949-62, ix.
Abstract Link:	http://www.medifocus.com/abstracts.php?gid=RH011&ID=18984414

19.

Issues related to clinical trials of oral and biologic disease-modifying agents for Sjogren's syndrome.

Author:	Carsons SE
Institution:	SUNY at Stony Brook School of Medicine, Stony Brook, NY, USA. Scarsons@winthrop.org
Journal:	Rheum Dis Clin North Am. 2008 Nov;34(4):1011-23, x.
Abstract Link:	http://www.medifocus.com/abstracts.php?gid=RH011&ID=18984419

Go to http://www.medifocus.com/links/RH011/0112 for direct online access to the above Abstract Links.

20.

Genes and Sjogren's syndrome.

Authors:	Cobb BL; Lessard CJ; Harley JB; Moser KL
Institution:	Arthritis and Immunology Program, Oklahoma Medical Research Foundation, 825 NE 13th Street, Oklahoma City, OK 73104, USA.
Journal:	Rheum Dis Clin North Am. 2008 Nov;34(4):847-68, vii.
Abstract Link:	http://www.medifocus.com/abstracts.php?gid=RH011&ID=18984408

21.

New concepts in the pathogenesis of Sjogren's syndrome.

Authors:	Delaleu N; Jonsson MV; Appel S; Jonsson R
Institution:	Broegelmann Research Laboratory, The Gade Institute, University of Bergen, Haukelandsveien 28, Bergen 5021, Norway.
Journal:	Rheum Dis Clin North Am. 2008 Nov;34(4):833-45, vii.
Abstract Link:	http://www.medifocus.com/abstracts.php?gid=RH011&ID=18984407

22.

Neuroelectrostimulation in treatment of hyposalivation and xerostomia in Sjogren's syndrome: a salivary pacemaker.

Authors:	Fedele S; Wolff A; Strietzel F; Lopez RM; Porter SR; Konttinen YT
Institution:	UCL Eastman Dental Institute, London, United Kingdom. s.fedele@eastman.ucl.ac.uk
Journal:	J Rheumatol. 2008 Aug;35(8):1489-94.
Abstract Link:	**ABSTRACT NOT AVAILABLE**

Go to http://www.medifocus.com/links/RH011/0112 for direct online access to the above Abstract Links.

23.

Treatment of dry eye disease by the non-ophthalmologist.

Author:	Foulks GN
Institution:	Department of Ophthalmology and Visual Sciences, University of Louisville School of Medicine, 301 East Muhammad Ali Boulevard, Louisville, KY 40202, USA. gnfoul01@louisville.edu
Journal:	Rheum Dis Clin North Am. 2008 Nov;34(4):987-1000, x.
Abstract Link:	http://www.medifocus.com/abstracts.php?gid=RH011&ID=18984417

24.

Anti-CD20 treatment in primary Sjogren's syndrome.

Authors:	Isaksen K; Jonsson R; Omdal R
Institution:	Department of Internal Medicine, Stavanger University Hospital, Stavanger, Norway. isak@sus.no
Journal:	Scand J Immunol. 2008 Dec;68(6):554-64. Epub 2008 Oct 23.
Abstract Link:	http://www.medifocus.com/abstracts.php?gid=RH011&ID=19000095

25.

Therapeutic potential for B-cell modulation in Sjogren's syndrome.

Author:	Mariette X
Institution:	Hopital Bicetre, Assistance Publique-Hopitaux de Paris (AP-HP), Universite Paris-Sud 11, Le Kremlin Bicetre, Institut Pour la Sante et la Recherche Medicale (INSERM) U 802, France. xavier.mariette@bct.aphp-paris.fr
Journal:	Rheum Dis Clin North Am. 2008 Nov;34(4):1025-33, x.
Abstract Link:	http://www.medifocus.com/abstracts.php?gid=RH011&ID=18984420

Go to http://www.medifocus.com/links/RH011/0112 for direct online access to the above Abstract Links.

26.

Oral manifestations of Sjogren's syndrome.

Authors:	Mathews SA; Kurien BT; Scofield RH
Institution:	University of Central Oklahoma, Edmond, OK, USA.
Journal:	J Dent Res. 2008 Apr;87(4):308-18.
Abstract Link:	http://www.medifocus.com/abstracts.php?gid=RH011&ID=18362310

27.

Treatment of central nervous system involvement associated with primary Sjogren's syndrome.

Authors:	Ozgocmen S; Gur A
Institution:	Division of Rheumatology, Department of Physical Medicine and Rehabilitation, Firat University, Faculty of Medicine, Elazig, Turkey. sozgocmen@hotmail.com
Journal:	Curr Pharm Des. 2008;14(13):1270-3.
Abstract Link:	http://www.medifocus.com/abstracts.php?gid=RH011&ID=18537651

28.

Pulmonary manifestations of primary Sjogren's syndrome.

Author:	Parke AL
Institution:	Division of Rheumatology, Saint Francis Hospital and Medical Center, 114 Woodland Street, Hartford, CT 06105-1208, USA.
Journal:	Rheum Dis Clin North Am. 2008 Nov;34(4):907-20, viii.
Abstract Link:	http://www.medifocus.com/abstracts.php?gid=RH011&ID=18984411

Go to http://www.medifocus.com/links/RH011/0112 for direct online access to the above Abstract Links.

29.

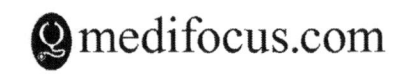

Hepatitis C virus and Sjogren's syndrome: trigger or mimic?

Authors: Ramos-Casals M; Munoz S; Zeron PB
Institution: Laboratory of Autoimmune Diseases "Josep Font," IDIBAPS, Department of Autoimmune Diseases, C/Villaroel 170, Hospital Clinic, Barcelona 08036, Spain. mramos@clinic.ub.es
Journal: Rheum Dis Clin North Am. 2008 Nov;34(4):869-84, vii.
Abstract Link: http://www.medifocus.com/abstracts.php?gid=RH011&ID=18984409

30.

Involvement of nervous system pathways in primary Sjogren's syndrome.

Authors: Segal B; Carpenter A; Walk D
Institution: Division of Rheumatic and Autoimmune Disorders, University of Minnesota Medical School, MMC 108, 420 Delaware SE, Minneapolis, MN 55455, USA. segal017@umn.edu
Journal: Rheum Dis Clin North Am. 2008 Nov;34(4):885-906, viii.
Abstract Link: http://www.medifocus.com/abstracts.php?gid=RH011&ID=18984410

31.

Sjogren's syndrome in childhood.

Authors: Singer NG; Tomanova-Soltys I; Lowe R
Institution: Division of Pediatric Infectious Diseases and Rheumatology, Rainbow Babies and Children's Hospital, Cleveland, OH 44106, USA. nora.singer@uhhospitals.org
Journal: Curr Rheumatol Rep. 2008 Apr;10(2):147-55.
Abstract Link: http://www.medifocus.com/abstracts.php?gid=RH011&ID=18460271

Go to http://www.medifocus.com/links/RH011/0112 for direct online access to the above Abstract Links.

32.

Primary Sjogren's syndrome: current and prospective therapies.

Authors:	Thanou-Stavraki A; James JA
Institution:	Arthritis and Immunology Program, Oklahoma Medical Research Foundation, Oklahoma City, Oklahoma 73104, USA.
Journal:	Semin Arthritis Rheum. 2008 Apr;37(5):273-92. Epub 2007 Aug 21.
Abstract Link:	http://www.medifocus.com/abstracts.php?gid=RH011&ID=17714766

33.

Relationship of Sjogren's syndrome to other connective tissue and autoimmune disorders.

Authors:	Theander E; Jacobsson LT
Institution:	Department of Rheumatology, Malmo University Hospital, Lund University, 20502 Malmo, Sweden. elke.theander@med.lu.se
Journal:	Rheum Dis Clin North Am. 2008 Nov;34(4):935-47, viii-ix.
Abstract Link:	http://www.medifocus.com/abstracts.php?gid=RH011&ID=18984413

34.

Neuroendocrine dysfunction in Sjogren's syndrome.

Authors:	Tzioufas AG; Tsonis J; Moutsopoulos HM
Institution:	Department of Pathophysiology, School of Medicine, University of Athens, Athens, Greece. agtzi@med.uoa.gr
Journal:	Neuroimmunomodulation. 2008;15(1):37-45. Epub 2008 Jul 29.
Abstract Link:	http://www.medifocus.com/abstracts.php?gid=RH011&ID=18667798

Go to http://www.medifocus.com/links/RH011/0112 for direct online access to the above Abstract Links.

35.

Measurement of disease activity and damage in Sjogren's syndrome.

Author:	Vitali C
Institution:	Department of Internal Medicine and Section of Rheumatology, 'Villamarina' Hospital, Piombino, Italy. c.vitali@yahoo.it
Journal:	Rheum Dis Clin North Am. 2008 Nov;34(4):963-71, ix.
Abstract Link:	http://www.medifocus.com/abstracts.php?gid=RH011&ID=18984415

36.

Role of nuclear scintigraphy in the characterization and management of the salivary component of Sjogren's syndrome.

Authors:	Vivino FB; Hermann GA
Institution:	Penn Presbyterian Medical Center, Penn Sjogren's Syndrome Center, University of Pennsylvania School of Medicine, 51 North 39th Street, 3910 Building, Philadelphia, PA 19104, USA. frederick.vivino@uphs.upenn.edu
Journal:	Rheum Dis Clin North Am. 2008 Nov;34(4):973-86, ix.
Abstract Link:	http://www.medifocus.com/abstracts.php?gid=RH011&ID=18984416

37.

Mucosa-associated lymphoid tissue lymphoma in Sjogren's syndrome: risks, management, and prognosis.

Authors:	Voulgarelis M; Moutsopoulos HM
Institution:	Department of Pathophysiology, Medical School, National University of Athens, 75 Mikras Asias Street, 11527 Athens, Greece. mvoulgar@med.uoa.gr
Journal:	Rheum Dis Clin North Am. 2008 Nov;34(4):921-33, viii.
Abstract Link:	http://www.medifocus.com/abstracts.php?gid=RH011&ID=18984412

Go to http://www.medifocus.com/links/RH011/0112 for direct online access to the above Abstract Links.

38.

Mortality in Sjogren's syndrome.

Authors:	Voulgarelis M; Tzioufas AG; Moutsopoulos HM
Institution:	Department of Pathophysiology, Medical School, National University of Athens, Greece.
Journal:	Clin Exp Rheumatol. 2008 Sep-Oct;26(5 Suppl 51):S66-71.
Abstract Link:	http://www.medifocus.com/abstracts.php?gid=RH011&ID=19026146

39.

Optimizing dry mouth treatment for individuals with Sjogren's syndrome.

Author:	Wu AJ
Institution:	Sjogren's Syndrome Clinic, University of California, San Francisco, 513 Parnassus Avenue, Room C646, CA 94143, USA. ava.wu@ucsf.edu
Journal:	Rheum Dis Clin North Am. 2008 Nov;34(4):1001-10, x.
Abstract Link:	http://www.medifocus.com/abstracts.php?gid=RH011&ID=18984418

Go to http://www.medifocus.com/links/RH011/0112 for direct online access to the above Abstract Links.

General Interest Articles

40.

Severe chronic bronchiolitis as the presenting feature of primary Sjogren's syndrome.

Authors:	Borie R; Schneider S; Debray MP; Adle-Biasssette H; Danel C; Bergeron A; Mariette X; Aubier M; Papo T; Crestani B
Institution:	Assistance Publique-Hopitaux de Paris, Hopital Bichat, Service de Pneumologie A, Centre de Competence maladies rares pulmonaires, Paris, France.
Journal:	Respir Med. 2011 Jan;105(1):130-6. Epub 2010 Nov 2.
Abstract Link:	http://www.medifocus.com/abstracts.php?gid=RH011&ID=21050739

41.

Elderly onset of primary Sjogren's syndrome: clinical manifestations, serological features and oral/ocular diagnostic tests. Comparison with adult and young onset of the disease in a cohort of 336 Italian patients.

Authors:	Botsios C; Furlan A; Ostuni P; Sfriso P; Andretta M; Ometto F; Raffeiner B; Todesco S; Punzi L
Institution:	Rheumatology Unit, Department of Clinical and Experimental Medicine, University of Padova, via Giustiniani 2, 35128 Padova, Italy. constantin.botsios@unipd.it
Journal:	Joint Bone Spine. 2011 Mar;78(2):171-4.
Abstract Link:	http://www.medifocus.com/abstracts.php?gid=RH011&ID=20620090

42.

The minimally important difference (MID) for patient-reported outcomes including pain, fatigue, sleep and the health assessment questionnaire disability index (HAQ-DI) in primary Sjogren's syndrome.

Authors:	George A; Pope JE
Institution:	Schulich School of Medicine, University of Western Ontario, London, Ontario, Canada.
Journal:	Clin Exp Rheumatol. 2011 Mar-Apr;29(2):248-53. Epub 2011 Apr 19.
Abstract Link:	http://www.medifocus.com/abstracts.php?gid=RH011&ID=21385542

Go to http://www.medifocus.com/links/RH011/0112 for direct online access to the above Abstract Links.

43.

Clinical manifestations of neurological involvement in primary Sjogren's syndrome.

Authors:	Gono T; Kawaguchi Y; Katsumata Y; Takagi K; Tochimoto A; Baba S; Okamoto Y; Ota Y; Yamanaka H
Institution:	Institute of Rheumatology, Tokyo Women's Medical University, 10-22 Kawada-cho, Shinjuku-Ku Tokyo 162-0054, Japan.
Journal:	Clin Rheumatol. 2011 Apr;30(4):485-90.
Abstract Link:	http://www.medifocus.com/abstracts.php?gid=RH011&ID=20393864

44.

The sparkle of the eye: the impact of ocular surface wetness on corneal light reflection.

Authors:	Goto E; Dogru M; Sato EA; Matsumoto Y; Takano Y; Tsubota K
Institution:	Department of Ophthalmology, School of Dental Medicine, Tsurumi University, 2-1-3 Tsurumi, Yokohama City, Kanagawa, Japan 230-8501. goto-e@tsurumi-u.ac.jp
Journal:	Am J Ophthalmol. 2011 Apr;151(4):691-696.e1. Epub 2011 Jan 21.
Abstract Link:	http://www.medifocus.com/abstracts.php?gid=RH011&ID=21255764

45.

Prevalence of IgA class antibodies to cyclic citrullinated peptide (anti-CCP) in patients with primary Sjogren's syndrome, and its association to clinical manifestations.

Authors:	Haga HJ; Andersen DT; Peen E
Institution:	Aalborg University Esbjerg, 6700 Esbjerg, Denmark. hjh@reumaklinikdanmark.dk
Journal:	Clin Rheumatol. 2011 Mar;30(3):369-72. Epub 2011 Jan 14.
Abstract Link:	http://www.medifocus.com/abstracts.php?gid=RH011&ID=21234630

Go to http://www.medifocus.com/links/RH011/0112 for direct online access to the above Abstract Links.

46.

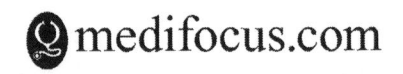

Two-year outcome of partial lacrimal punctal occlusion in the management of dry eye related to Sjogren syndrome.

Authors:	Holzchuh R; Villa Albers MB; Osaki TH; Igami TZ; Santo RM; Kara-Jose N; Holzchuh N; Hida RY
Institution:	Department of Ophthalmology, Hospital das Clinicas of University of Sao Paulo, Brazil.
Journal:	Curr Eye Res. 2011 Jun;36(6):507-12.
Abstract Link:	http://www.medifocus.com/abstracts.php?gid=RH011&ID=21591859

47.

Pregnancy and fetal outcome in women with primary Sjogren's syndrome compared with women in the general population: a nested case-control study.

Authors:	Hussein SZ; Jacobsson LT; Lindquist PG; Theander E
Institution:	Department of Rheumatology, Lund University, Skane University Hospital, Malmo, Sweden.
Journal:	Rheumatology (Oxford). 2011 Sep;50(9):1612-7. Epub 2011 Apr 29.
Abstract Link:	http://www.medifocus.com/abstracts.php?gid=RH011&ID=21531959

48.

The psychological defensive profile of primary Sjogren's syndrome patients and its relationship to health-related quality of life.

Authors:	Hyphantis T; Mantis D; Voulgari PV; Tsifetaki N; Drosos AA
Institution:	Department of Psychiatry, Medical School, University of Ioannina, Ioannina, Greece.
Journal:	Clin Exp Rheumatol. 2011 May-Jun;29(3):485-93. Epub 2011 Jun 29.
Abstract Link:	http://www.medifocus.com/abstracts.php?gid=RH011&ID=21640041

Go to http://www.medifocus.com/links/RH011/0112 for direct online access to the above Abstract Links.

49.

Anxiety and depression in patients with dry eye syndrome.

Authors:	Li M; Gong L; Sun X; Chapin WJ
Institution:	Department of Ophthalmology, EYE & ENT Hospital of Fudan University, No. 83 Fenyang Road, Shanghai, China.
Journal:	Curr Eye Res. 2011 Jan;36(1):1-7.
Abstract Link:	http://www.medifocus.com/abstracts.php?gid=RH011&ID=21174591

50.

Atypical neurologic complications in patients with primary Sjogren's syndrome: report of 4 cases.

Authors:	Michel L; Toulgoat F; Desal H; Laplaud DA; Magot A; Hamidou M; Wiertlewski S
Institution:	Service de Neurologie, Centre Hospitalier Universitaire de Nantes, Hopital Laennec, Nantes Cedex, France. Laure.michel@univ-nantes.fr
Journal:	Semin Arthritis Rheum. 2011 Feb;40(4):338-42. Epub 2010 Aug 10.
Abstract Link:	http://www.medifocus.com/abstracts.php?gid=RH011&ID=20701954

51.

Peripheral neuropathies in Sjogren syndrome: a new reappraisal.

Authors:	Pavlakis PP; Alexopoulos H; Kosmidis ML; Stamboulis E; Routsias JG; Tzartos SJ; Tzioufas AG; Moutsopoulos HM; Dalakas MC
Institution:	Department of Pathophysiology, Medical School, University of Athens, Athens, Greece.
Journal:	J Neurol Neurosurg Psychiatry. 2011 Jul;82(7):798-802. Epub 2010 Dec 16.
Abstract Link:	http://www.medifocus.com/abstracts.php?gid=RH011&ID=21172862

Go to http://www.medifocus.com/links/RH011/0112 for direct online access to the above Abstract Links.

52.

Novel carbonic anhydrase autoantibodies and renal manifestations in patients with primary Sjogren's syndrome.

Authors:	Pertovaara M; Bootorabi F; Kuuslahti M; Pasternack A; Parkkila S
Institution:	Department of Internal Medicine, Rheumatology Centre, Tampere University Hospital, Tampere, Finland. marja.pertovaara@uta.fi
Journal:	Rheumatology (Oxford). 2011 Aug;50(8):1453-7. Epub 2011 Mar 22.
Abstract Link:	http://www.medifocus.com/abstracts.php?gid=RH011&ID=21427176

53.

Peripheral neuropathies associated with primary Sjogren syndrome: immunologic profiles of nonataxic sensory neuropathy and sensorimotor neuropathy.

Authors:	Sene D; Jallouli M; Lefaucheur JP; Saadoun D; Costedoat-Chalumeau N; Maisonobe T; Diemert MC; Musset L; Haroche J; Piette JC; Amoura Z; Cacoub P
Institution:	Service de Medecine Interne, AP-HP, Hopital Pitie-Salpetriere, and Universite Pierre et Marie Curie-Paris 6, Paris, France. damien.sene@psl.aphp.fr
Journal:	Medicine (Baltimore). 2011 Mar;90(2):133-8.
Abstract Link:	http://www.medifocus.com/abstracts.php?gid=RH011&ID=21358442

54.

Endoscopic treatment of salivary glands affected by autoimmune diseases.

Authors:	Shacham R; Puterman MB; Ohana N; Nahlieli O
Institution:	Department of Oral and Maxillofacial Surgery, Barzilai Medical Center, Ashkelon, Israel.
Journal:	J Oral Maxillofac Surg. 2011 Feb;69(2):476-81. Epub 2010 Dec 8.
Abstract Link:	http://www.medifocus.com/abstracts.php?gid=RH011&ID=21145154

Go to http://www.medifocus.com/links/RH011/0112 for direct online access to the above Abstract Links.

55.

Relation of systemic autoantibodies to the number of extraglandular manifestations in primary Sjogren's Syndrome: a retrospective analysis of 65 patients in the Netherlands.

Authors:	ter Borg EJ; Risselada AP; Kelder JC
Institution:	Department of Rheumatology, St. Antonius Hospital, Nieuwegein, The Netherlands. borg@antoniusziekenhuis.nl
Journal:	Semin Arthritis Rheum. 2011 Jun;40(6):547-51. doi: 10.1016/j.semarthrit.2010.07.006. Epub 2010 Sep 22.
Abstract Link:	http://www.medifocus.com/abstracts.php?gid=RH011&ID=20864144

56.

Long-term use of hydroxypropyl cellulose ophthalmic insert to relieve symptoms of dry eye in a contact lens wearer: case-based experience.

Author:	Wander AH
Institution:	Department of Ophthalmology, University of Cincinnati College of Medicine and Academic Health Center, Cincinnati, OH, USA. myersdo@ucphysicians.com
Journal:	Eye Contact Lens. 2011 Jan;37(1):39-44.
Abstract Link:	http://www.medifocus.com/abstracts.php?gid=RH011&ID=21178699

57.

Hydroxychloroquine improves dry eye symptoms of patients with primary Sjogren's syndrome.

Authors:	Yavuz S; Asfuroglu E; Bicakcigil M; Toker E
Institution:	Department of Rheumatology, Marmara University Medical School, Istanbul, Turkey. suleyavuz@gmail.com
Journal:	Rheumatol Int. 2011 Aug;31(8):1045-9. Epub 2010 Mar 23.
Abstract Link:	http://www.medifocus.com/abstracts.php?gid=RH011&ID=20309693

Go to http://www.medifocus.com/links/RH011/0112 for direct online access to the above Abstract Links.

58.

Proceedings of the 10th International Symposium on Sjogren's Syndrome. October 1-3, 2009. Brest, France.

Author:	
Journal:	Autoimmun Rev. 2010 Jul;9(9):589-633.
Abstract Link:	**ABSTRACT NOT AVAILABLE**

59.

Acute motor axonal neuropathy in association with Sjogren syndrome.

Authors:	Awad A; Mathew S; Katirji B
Institution:	Neurological Institute, University Hospitals Case Medical Center, Case Western Reserve University, Cleveland, Ohio 44104, USA. ameraldo@gmail.com
Journal:	Muscle Nerve. 2010 Nov;42(5):828-30.
Abstract Link:	http://www.medifocus.com/abstracts.php?gid=RH011&ID=20976785

60.

Secondary Sjogren's syndrome in systemic lupus erythematosus defines a distinct disease subset.

Authors:	Baer AN; Maynard JW; Shaikh F; Magder LS; Petri M
Institution:	Division of Rheumatology, Good Samaritan Hospital, Russell Morgan Building, Suite 508, 5601 Loch Raven Blvd., Baltimore, MD 21239, USA. alanbaer@jhmi.edu
Journal:	J Rheumatol. 2010 Jun;37(6):1143-9. Epub 2010 Apr 1.
Abstract Link:	http://www.medifocus.com/abstracts.php?gid=RH011&ID=20360189

Go to http://www.medifocus.com/links/RH011/0112 for direct online access to the above Abstract Links.

61.

Impaired gastric emptying in primary Sjogren's syndrome.

Authors:	Hammar O; Ohlsson B; Wollmer P; Mandl T
Institution:	Department of Clinical Sciences, Division of Gastroenterology and Hepatology, Skane University Hospital, Lund University, Malmo, Sweden. oskar.hammar@med.lu.se
Journal:	J Rheumatol. 2010 Nov;37(11):2313-8. Epub 2010 Sep 1.
Abstract Link:	http://www.medifocus.com/abstracts.php?gid=RH011&ID=20810502

62.

Similarities and differences between primary and secondary Sjogren's syndrome.

Authors:	Hernandez-Molina G; Avila-Casado C; Cardenas-Velazquez F; Hernandez-Hernandez C; Calderillo ML; Marroquin V; Soto-Abraham V; Recillas-Gispert C; Sanchez-Guerrero J
Institution:	Department of Immunology and Rheumatology, Ophthalmology Service, and Dental Service, Instituto Nacional de Ciencias Medicas y Nutricion Salvador Zubiran, Mexico City, Mexico.
Journal:	J Rheumatol. 2010 Apr;37(4):800-8. Epub 2010 Mar 1.
Abstract Link:	http://www.medifocus.com/abstracts.php?gid=RH011&ID=20194453

63.

Evaluation of quality of life in relation to anxiety and depression in primary Sjogren's syndrome.

Authors:	Inal V; Kitapcioglu G; Karabulut G; Keser G; Kabasakal Y
Institution:	Division of Rheumatology, Department of Internal Medicine, Ege University School of Medicine, Izmir, Turkey.
Journal:	Mod Rheumatol. 2010 Dec;20(6):588-97. Epub 2010 Jun 29.
Abstract Link:	http://www.medifocus.com/abstracts.php?gid=RH011&ID=20585824

Go to http://www.medifocus.com/links/RH011/0112 for direct online access to the above Abstract Links.

64.

Comorbidities in patients with primary Sjogren's syndrome: a registry-based case-control study.

Authors:	Kang JH; Lin HC
Institution:	Department of Physical Medicine and Rehabilitation and Neuroscience Research Center, Taipei, Taiwan.
Journal:	J Rheumatol. 2010 Jun;37(6):1188-94. Epub 2010 Apr 1.
Abstract Link:	http://www.medifocus.com/abstracts.php?gid=RH011&ID=20360180

65.

Psychopathological and personality features in primary Sjogren's syndrome--associations with autoantibodies to neuropeptides.

Authors:	Karaiskos D; Mavragani CP; Sinno MH; Dechelotte P; Zintzaras E; Skopouli FN; Fetissov SO; Moutsopoulos HM
Institution:	Department of Pathophysiology, School of Medicine, University of Athens, Athens, Greece.
Journal:	Rheumatology (Oxford). 2010 Sep;49(9):1762-9. Epub 2010 Jun 4.
Abstract Link:	http://www.medifocus.com/abstracts.php?gid=RH011&ID=20525741

66.

Annular erythema associated with Sjogren's syndrome: review of the literature on the management and clinical analysis of skin lesions.

Authors:	Katayama I; Kotobuki Y; Kiyohara E; Murota H
Institution:	Department of Dermatology, Course of Integrated Medicine, Graduate School of Medicine, Osaka University, 2-2 Yamada-oka, Suita, Osaka, 565-0871, Japan, katayama@derma.med.Osaka-u.ac.jp.
Journal:	Mod Rheumatol. 2010 Jan 8.
Abstract Link:	http://www.medifocus.com/abstracts.php?gid=RH011&ID=20054701

Go to http://www.medifocus.com/links/RH011/0112 for direct online access to the above Abstract Links.

67.

Is there progressive cognitive dysfunction in Sjogren Syndrome? A preliminary study.

Authors:	Martinez S; Caceres C; Mataro M; Escudero D; Latorre P; Davalos A
Institution:	Neurology Department, Hospital Universitari Germans Trias i Pujol, Badalona, Spain.
Journal:	Acta Neurol Scand. 2010 Sep;122(3):182-8. Epub 2010 Jan 21.
Abstract Link:	http://www.medifocus.com/abstracts.php?gid=RH011&ID=20096020

68.

Cardiovascular risk factors in primary Sjogren's syndrome: a case-control study in 624 patients.

Authors:	Perez-De-Lis M; Akasbi M; Siso A; Diez-Cascon P; Brito-Zeron P; Diaz-Lagares C; Ortiz J; Perez-Alvarez R; Ramos-Casals M; Coca A
Institution:	Sjogren Syndrome Research Group (AGAUR), Laboratory of Autoimmune Diseases Josep Font, Institut d'Investigacions Biomediques August Pi i Sunyer, Department of Autoimmune Diseases, Barcelona, Spain.
Journal:	Lupus. 2010 Jul;19(8):941-8.
Abstract Link:	http://www.medifocus.com/abstracts.php?gid=RH011&ID=20581017

69.

Fatigue in Sjogren's syndrome: relationship with fibromyalgia, clinical and biologic features.

Authors:	Priori R; Iannuccelli C; Alessandri C; Modesti M; Antonazzo B; Di Lollo AC; Valesini G; Di Franco M
Institution:	Dipartimento di Medicina Interna e Specialita Mediche, Reumatologia, Universita La Sapienza, Rome, Italy. rob.pri@libero.it
Journal:	Clin Exp Rheumatol. 2010 Nov-Dec;28(6 Suppl 63):S82-6. Epub 2010 Dec 22.
Abstract Link:	http://www.medifocus.com/abstracts.php?gid=RH011&ID=21176426

Go to http://www.medifocus.com/links/RH011/0112 for direct online access to the above Abstract Links.

70.

Clinical and Prognostic Significance of Parotid Scintigraphy in 405 Patients with Primary Sjogren's Syndrome.

Authors:	Ramos-Casals M; Brito-Zeron P; Perez-De-Lis M; Diaz-Lagares C; Bove A; Soto MJ; Jimenez I; Belenguer R; Siso A; Muxi A; Pons F
Institution:	From the Sjogren Syndrome Research Group (AGAUR), Laboratory of Autoimmune Diseases Josep Font, IDIBAPS, Department of Autoimmune Diseases; Nuclear Medicine Department (Centre de Diagnostic per la Imatge); CAP Les Corts, GESCLINIC, Hospital Clinic, Barcelona; and Rheumatology Unit, Hospital 9 d'Octubre, Valencia, Spain.
Journal:	J Rheumatol. 2010 Jan 15.
Abstract Link:	http://www.medifocus.com/abstracts.php?gid=RH011&ID=20080906

71.

Effects of Reduced Saliva Production on Swallowing in Patients with Sjogren's Syndrome.

Authors:	Rogus-Pulia NM; Logemann JA
Institution:	Department of Communication Sciences and Disorders, Northwestern University, Evanston, IL, 60208-3570, USA, nicoleroguspulia@gmail.com.
Journal:	Dysphagia. 2010 Oct 28.
Abstract Link:	http://www.medifocus.com/abstracts.php?gid=RH011&ID=20981451

72.

EULAR Sjogren's syndrome disease activity index: development of a consensus systemic disease activity index for primary Sjogren's syndrome.

Authors:	Seror R; Ravaud P; Bowman SJ; Baron G; Tzioufas A; Theander E; Gottenberg JE; Bootsma H; Mariette X; Vitali C
Institution:	Department of Epidemiology, Biostatistics and Clinical Research, Hopital Bichat, INSERM U738, Hopital Bichat, 46 rue Henri Huchard, Paris 75018, France. raphaele.se@gmail.com
Journal:	Ann Rheum Dis. 2010 Jun;69(6):1103-9. Epub 2009 Jun 28.
Abstract Link:	http://www.medifocus.com/abstracts.php?gid=RH011&ID=19561361

Go to http://www.medifocus.com/links/RH011/0112 for direct online access to the above Abstract Links.

73.

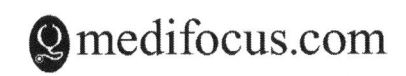

Effect of omega-3 and vitamin E supplementation on dry mouth in patients with Sjogren's syndrome.

Authors:	Singh M; Stark PC; Palmer CA; Gilbard JP; Papas AS
Institution:	Division of Oral Medicine and Dental Research, Tufts University School of Dental Medicine, Boston, Massachusetts, USA. periodok@yahoo.com
Journal:	Spec Care Dentist. 2010 Nov-Dec;30(6):225-9. doi: 10.1111/j.1754-4505.2010.00158.x. Epub 2010 Oct 19.
Abstract Link:	http://www.medifocus.com/abstracts.php?gid=RH011&ID=21044101

74.

Bronchiectasis in primary Sjogren's syndrome: prevalence and clinical significance.

Authors:	Soto-Cardenas MJ; Perez-De-Lis M; Bove A; Navarro C; Brito-Zeron P; Diaz-Lagares C; Gandia M; Akasbi M; Siso A; Ballester E; Torres A; Ramos-Casals M
Institution:	Sjogren's Syndrome Research Group (AGAUR), Laboratory of Autoimmune Diseases Josep Font, IDIBAPS, Department of Autoimmune Diseases, Hospital Clinic, Barcelona, Spain. mariajose.soto@uca.es
Journal:	Clin Exp Rheumatol. 2010 Sep-Oct;28(5):647-53. Epub 2010 Oct 22.
Abstract Link:	http://www.medifocus.com/abstracts.php?gid=RH011&ID=20883638

75.

Variability of fatigue during the day in patients with primary Sjogren's syndrome, systemic lupus erythematosus, and rheumatoid arthritis.

Authors:	van Oers ML; Bossema ER; Thoolen BJ; Hartkamp A; Dekkers JC; Godaert GL; Kruize AA; Derksen RH; Bijlsma JW; Geenen R
Institution:	Department of Clinical and Health Psychology, Utrecht University, Utrecht, The Netherlands. marijnvanoers@gmail.com
Journal:	Clin Exp Rheumatol. 2010 Sep-Oct;28(5):715-21. Epub 2010 Oct 22.
Abstract Link:	http://www.medifocus.com/abstracts.php?gid=RH011&ID=20863446

Go to http://www.medifocus.com/links/RH011/0112 for direct online access to the above Abstract Links.

76.

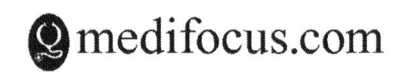

Sjogren's syndrome-onset lupus patients have distinctive clinical manifestations and benign prognosis: a case-control study.

Authors:	Xu D; Tian X; Zhang W; Zhang X; Liu B; Zhang F
Institution:	Department of Rheumatology, Peking Union Medical College (PUMC) Hospital, Chinese Academy of Medical Sciences and Peking Union Medical College, Beijing 100730, China.
Journal:	Lupus. 2010 Feb;19(2):197-200. Epub 2009 Nov 9.
Abstract Link:	http://www.medifocus.com/abstracts.php?gid=RH011&ID=19900977

77.

Lung involvement in patients with primary Sjogren's syndrome: what are the predictors?

Authors:	Yazisiz V; Arslan G; Ozbudak IH; Turker S; Erbasan F; Avci AB; Ozbudak O; Terzioglu E
Institution:	Division of Rheumatology and Immunology, Department of Internal Medicine, Akdeniz Universitesi Tip Fakultesi Ic Hastaliklari AD, Antalya, Turkey. drvyazisiz@yahoo.com.tr
Journal:	Rheumatol Int. 2010 Aug;30(10):1317-24. Epub 2009 Oct 21.
Abstract Link:	http://www.medifocus.com/abstracts.php?gid=RH011&ID=19844720

78.

Evaluation of patients with dry eye for presence of underlying Sjogren syndrome.

Authors:	Akpek EK; Klimava A; Thorne JE; Martin D; Lekhanont K; Ostrovsky A
Institution:	Ocular Surface Diseases and Dry Eye Clinic, Division of Cornea, Wilmer Eye Institute, The Johns Hopkins University School of Medicine, Baltimore, MD, USA. esakpek@jhmi.edu
Journal:	Cornea. 2009 Jun;28(5):493-7.
Abstract Link:	http://www.medifocus.com/abstracts.php?gid=RH011&ID=19421051

Go to http://www.medifocus.com/links/RH011/0112 for direct online access to the above Abstract Links.

79.

Periodontal conditions of individuals with Sjogren's syndrome.

Authors:	Antoniazzi RP; Miranda LA; Zanatta FB; Islabao AG; Gustafsson A; Chiapinotto GA; Oppermann RV
Institution:	Postgraduate Program in Dentistry, Brazilian Lutheran University, Canoas, RS, Brazil. raquelantoniazzi@hotmail.com
Journal:	J Periodontol. 2009 Mar;80(3):429-35.
Abstract Link:	http://www.medifocus.com/abstracts.php?gid=RH011&ID=19254127

80.

Hematologic manifestations and predictors of lymphoma development in primary Sjogren syndrome: clinical and pathophysiologic aspects.

Authors:	Baimpa E; Dahabreh IJ; Voulgarelis M; Moutsopoulos HM
Institution:	Department of Pathophysiology, Medical School of Athens, National University of Athens, Athens, Greece.
Journal:	Medicine (Baltimore). 2009 Sep;88(5):284-93.
Abstract Link:	http://www.medifocus.com/abstracts.php?gid=RH011&ID=19745687

81.

The minor salivary gland biopsy as a diagnostic tool for Sjogren syndrome.

Authors:	Bamba R; Sweiss NJ; Langerman AJ; Taxy JB; Blair EA
Institution:	Pritzker School of Medicine, University of Chicago, Chicago, Illinois, U.S.A.
Journal:	Laryngoscope. 2009 Oct;119(10):1922-6.
Abstract Link:	http://www.medifocus.com/abstracts.php?gid=RH011&ID=19650134

82.

Emerging Treatment Strategies and Potential Therapeutic Targets in Primary Sjogren's Syndrome.

Authors:	Becker H; Pavenstaedt H; Willeke P
Institution:	Department of Medicine D, University of Muenster, Muenster, Germany. beckerhe@mednet.uni-muenster.de.
Journal:	Inflamm Allergy Drug Targets. 2009 Sep 1.
Abstract Link:	http://www.medifocus.com/abstracts.php?gid=RH011&ID=19906008

83.

Patient-reported outcomes in primary Sjogren's syndrome: comparison of the long and short versions of the Profile of Fatigue and Discomfort--Sicca Symptoms Inventory.

Authors:	Bowman SJ; Hamburger J; Richards A; Barry RJ; Rauz S
Institution:	Department of Rheumatology, University Hospital Birmingham NHS Foundation Trust (Selly Oak), Raddlebarn Road, Birmingham B296JD, UK. simon.bowman@uhb.nhs.uk
Journal:	Rheumatology (Oxford). 2009 Feb;48(2):140-3. Epub 2008 Dec 11.
Abstract Link:	http://www.medifocus.com/abstracts.php?gid=RH011&ID=19074185

84.

B cell depletion in lupus and Sjogren's syndrome: an update.

Authors:	Coca A; Sanz I
Institution:	Division of Allergy, Immunology and Rheumatology, University of Rochester, Rochester, New York 14642, USA.
Journal:	Curr Opin Rheumatol. 2009 Sep;21(5):483-8.
Abstract Link:	http://www.medifocus.com/abstracts.php?gid=RH011&ID=19644378

Go to http://www.medifocus.com/links/RH011/0112 for direct online access to the above Abstract Links.

85.

B-cell-directed therapies for autoimmune disease.

Authors:	Dorner T; Radbruch A; Burmester GR
Institution:	Charite Center 12 and 14, Charite University Hospital & Deutsches Rheuma-Forschungszentrum Berlin, Berlin, Germany. thomas.doerner@charite.de
Journal:	Nat Rev Rheumatol. 2009 Aug;5(8):433-41. Epub 2009 Jul 7.
Abstract Link:	http://www.medifocus.com/abstracts.php?gid=RH011&ID=19581902

86.

Minor salivary gland biopsy to detect primary Sjogren syndrome in patients with interstitial lung disease.

Authors:	Fischer A; Swigris JJ; du Bois RM; Groshong SD; Cool CD; Sahin H; Lynch DA; Gillis JZ; Cohen MD; Meehan RT; Brown KK
Institution:	Autoimmune and Interstitial Lung Disease Program, Department of Medicine, National Jewish Health, 1400 Jackson St, Denver, CO 80206, USA. fischera@njhealth.org
Journal:	Chest. 2009 Oct;136(4):1072-8. Epub 2009 May 8.
Abstract Link:	http://www.medifocus.com/abstracts.php?gid=RH011&ID=19429722

87.

Epidemiological studies in incidence, prevalence, mortality, and comorbidity of the rheumatic diseases.

Authors:	Gabriel SE; Michaud K
Institution:	Department of Health Sciences Research, Mayo Foundation, Rochester, MN 55905, USA. gabriel.sherine@mayo.edu
Journal:	Arthritis Res Ther. 2009;11(3):229. Epub 2009 May 19.
Abstract Link:	http://www.medifocus.com/abstracts.php?gid=RH011&ID=19519924

Go to http://www.medifocus.com/links/RH011/0112 for direct online access to the above Abstract Links.

88.

Diagnostic evaluation and classification criteria in Sjogren's Syndrome.

Authors:	Galvez J; Saiz E; Lopez P; Pina MF; Carrillo A; Nieto A; Perez A; Marras C; Linares LF; Tornero C; Climent A; Rosique J; Reyes Y
Institution:	Rheumatology Unit, Hospital General Universitario JM Morales Meseguer, C/ Marques de los Velez s/n, Murcia 30008, Spain. ppgalvis@hotmail.com
Journal:	Joint Bone Spine. 2009 Jan;76(1):44-9. Epub 2008 Sep 30.
Abstract Link:	http://www.medifocus.com/abstracts.php?gid=RH011&ID=18829369

89.

Primary Sjogren's syndrome: pathophysiological, clinical and therapeutic advances.

Author:	Gottenberg JE
Institution:	Service de rhumatologie, centre national de reference pour les maladies auto-immunes systemiques rares, hopitaux universitaires de Strasbourg, 1, avenue Moliere, 67000 Strasbourg, France. jacques-eric.gottenberg@chru-strasbourg.fr
Journal:	Joint Bone Spine. 2009 Dec;76(6):591-4. Epub .
Abstract Link:	http://www.medifocus.com/abstracts.php?gid=RH011&ID=19932634

90.

The minor salivary gland proteome in Sjogren's syndrome.

Authors:	Hjelmervik TO; Jonsson R; Bolstad AI
Institution:	Department of Clinical Dentistry - Periodontics, University of Bergen, Bergen, Norway.
Journal:	Oral Dis. 2009 Jul;15(5):342-53. Epub 2009 Apr 2.
Abstract Link:	http://www.medifocus.com/abstracts.php?gid=RH011&ID=19364392

Go to http://www.medifocus.com/links/RH011/0112 for direct online access to the above Abstract Links.

91.

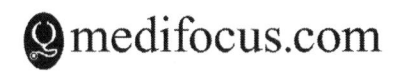

An experiment of the combined treatment of traditional Lei-huo-jiu therapy with Chinese medicine for the lacrimal gland of Sjogren's syndrome.

Authors:	Jin M; Song H; Pan L
Journal:	J Ocul Biol Dis Infor. 2009 Jun;2(2):65-72. Epub 2009 Jul 21.
Abstract Link:	http://www.medifocus.com/abstracts.php?gid=RH011&ID=19672465

92.

Impact of primary Sjogren's syndrome on smell and taste: effect on quality of life.

Authors:	Kamel UF; Maddison P; Whitaker R
Institution:	North West Wales NHS Trust, Bangor University, Bangor, UK.
Journal:	Rheumatology (Oxford). 2009 Dec;48(12):1512-4. Epub 2009 Sep 14.
Abstract Link:	http://www.medifocus.com/abstracts.php?gid=RH011&ID=19752179

93.

Secondary tumours in Sjogren's syndrome.

Authors:	Kovacs L; Szodoray P; Kiss E
Institution:	Department of Rheumatology, Albert Szent-Gyorgyi Clinical Centre, University of Szeged, Hungary.
Journal:	Autoimmun Rev. 2009 Jul 12.
Abstract Link:	http://www.medifocus.com/abstracts.php?gid=RH011&ID=19602455

Go to http://www.medifocus.com/links/RH011/0112 for direct online access to the above Abstract Links.

94.

Diagnosis and management of Sjogren syndrome.

Authors:	Kruszka P; O'Brian RJ
Institution:	U.S. Coast Guard Yard, Baltimore, Maryland, USA. paul_kruszka@hotmail.com
Journal:	Am Fam Physician. 2009 Mar 15;79(6):465-70.
Abstract Link:	http://www.medifocus.com/abstracts.php?gid=RH011&ID=19323359

95.

Chronic hepatitis B virus infection in Sjogren's syndrome. Prevalence and clinical significance in 603 patients.

Authors:	Marcos M; Alvarez F; Brito-Zeron P; Bove A; Perez-De-Lis M; Diaz-Lagares C; Sanchez-Tapias JM; Ramos-Casals M
Institution:	Department of Autoimmune Diseases, Institut d'Investigacions Biomediques August Pi i Sunyer (IDIBAPS), Hospital Clinic, Barcelona, Spain.
Journal:	Autoimmun Rev. 2009 Jun;8(7):616-20. Epub 2009 Feb 12.
Abstract Link:	http://www.medifocus.com/abstracts.php?gid=RH011&ID=19393197

96.

Sjogren's syndrome of the oral cavity. Review and update.

Authors:	Margaix-Munoz M; Bagan JV; Poveda R; Jimenez Y; Sarrion G
Institution:	Hospital General Universitario, Servicio de Estomatologia, Avda. Tres Cruces s/n, 46014 Valencia, Spain,margaix1980@hotmail.com.
Journal:	Med Oral Patol Oral Cir Bucal. 2009 Jul 1;14(7):E325-30.
Abstract Link:	http://www.medifocus.com/abstracts.php?gid=RH011&ID=19300364

Go to http://www.medifocus.com/links/RH011/0112 for direct online access to the above Abstract Links.

97.

Renal involvement in primary Sjogren's syndrome: a clinicopathologic study.

Authors:	Maripuri S; Grande JP; Osborn TG; Fervenza FC; Matteson EL; Donadio JV; Hogan MC
Institution:	Department of Internal Medicine, Mayo Clinic, Rochester, Minnesota 55905, USA.
Journal:	Clin J Am Soc Nephrol. 2009 Sep;4(9):1423-31. Epub 2009 Aug 13.
Abstract Link:	http://www.medifocus.com/abstracts.php?gid=RH011&ID=19679669

98.

Health-related quality of life, employment and disability in patients with Sjogren's syndrome.

Authors:	Meijer JM; Meiners PM; Huddleston Slater JJ; Spijkervet FK; Kallenberg CG; Vissink A; Bootsma H
Institution:	Department of Oral and Maxillofacial Surgery, University Medical Center Groningen, Groningen, The Netherlands.
Journal:	Rheumatology (Oxford). 2009 Sep;48(9):1077-82. Epub 2009 Jun 24.
Abstract Link:	http://www.medifocus.com/abstracts.php?gid=RH011&ID=19553376

99.

Association of severe inflammatory polyarthritis in primary Sjogren's syndrome: clinical, serologic, and HLA analysis.

Authors:	Mohammed K; Pope J; Le Riche N; Brintnell W; Cairns E; Coles R; Bell DA
Institution:	Department of Medicine, Division of Rheumatology, St Joseph's Health Care London and University of Western Ontario, London, Ontario, Canada.
Journal:	J Rheumatol. 2009 Sep;36(9):1937-42. Epub 2009 Jun 1.
Abstract Link:	http://www.medifocus.com/abstracts.php?gid=RH011&ID=19487261

Go to http://www.medifocus.com/links/RH011/0112 for direct online access to the above Abstract Links.

100.

Intravenous immunoglobulin treatment for painful sensory neuropathy associated with Sjogren's syndrome.

Authors:	Morozumi S; Kawagashira Y; Iijima M; Koike H; Hattori N; Katsuno M; Tanaka F; Sobue G
Institution:	Department of Neurology, Nagoya University Graduate School of Medicine, Nagoya, Japan.
Journal:	J Neurol Sci. 2009 Apr 15;279(1-2):57-61. Epub 2009 Jan 24.
Abstract Link:	http://www.medifocus.com/abstracts.php?gid=RH011&ID=19168191

101.

Pathogenesis of Sjogren's syndrome.

Authors:	Nikolov NP; Illei GG
Institution:	Sjogren's Syndrome Clinic, National Institute of Dental and Craniofacial Research (NIDCR), Molecular Physiology and Therapeutics Branch, National Institutes of Health (NIH), Bethesda, Maryland 20892, USA.
Journal:	Curr Opin Rheumatol. 2009 Sep;21(5):465-70.
Abstract Link:	http://www.medifocus.com/abstracts.php?gid=RH011&ID=19568172

102.

IgA rheumatoid factor in primary Sjogren's syndrome.

Authors:	Peen E; Mellbye OJ; Haga HJ
Institution:	Aalborg University Esbjerg, Esbjerg, Denmark.
Journal:	Scand J Rheumatol. 2009 Jan-Feb;38(1):46-9.
Abstract Link:	http://www.medifocus.com/abstracts.php?gid=RH011&ID=18942022

Go to http://www.medifocus.com/links/RH011/0112 for direct online access to the above Abstract Links.

103.

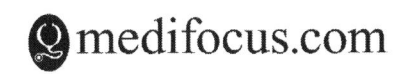

Prevalence of abnormal ankle brachial index in patients with primary Sjogren's syndrome.

Authors:	Rachapalli SM; Kiely PD; Bourke BE
Institution:	St George's Hospital, Blackshaw Road, Tooting, London, UK. satishmohanreddy@yahoo.com
Journal:	Clin Rheumatol. 2009 May;28(5):587-90. Epub 2009 Feb 10.
Abstract Link:	http://www.medifocus.com/abstracts.php?gid=RH011&ID=19205787

104.

Cytokines in Sjogren's syndrome.

Authors:	Roescher N; Tak PP; Illei GG
Institution:	Molecular Physiology and Therapeutics Branch, National Institute of Dental and Craniofacial Research, National Institutes of Health, DHHS, Bethesda, MD, USA.
Journal:	Oral Dis. 2009 Nov;15(8):519-26. Epub 2009 Jun 10.
Abstract Link:	http://www.medifocus.com/abstracts.php?gid=RH011&ID=19519622

105.

Primary Sjogren's Syndrome: health experiences and predictors of health quality among patients in the United States.

Authors:	Segal B; Bowman SJ; Fox PC; Vivino FB; Murukutla N; Brodscholl J; Ogale S; McLean L
Institution:	Associate Professor, Division of Rheumatic and Autoimmune Diseases, Department of Medicine, University of Minnesota, USA. segal017@umn.edu
Journal:	Health Qual Life Outcomes. 2009 May 27;7:46.
Abstract Link:	http://www.medifocus.com/abstracts.php?gid=RH011&ID=19473510

Go to http://www.medifocus.com/links/RH011/0112 for direct online access to the above Abstract Links.

106.

Pulmonary Manifestations of Sjogren's Syndrome.

Authors:	Shi JH; Liu HR; Xu WB; Feng RE; Zhang ZH; Tian XL; Zhu YJ
Institution:	Department of Pulmonary Medicine, Peking Union Medical College Hospital, Chinese Academy of Medical Science and Peking Union Medical College, Beijing, China.
Journal:	Respiration. 2009 Apr 22.
Abstract Link:	http://www.medifocus.com/abstracts.php?gid=RH011&ID=19390161

107.

B cell-targeted therapies in Sjogren's syndrome.

Authors:	Tobon GJ; Pers JO; Youinou P; Saraux A
Institution:	EA2216, IFR148, Universite de Bretagne Occidentale, Brest, France; Service de Rhumatologie, Centre Hospitalier Universitaire de Brest, Brest, France.
Journal:	Autoimmun Rev. 2009 Aug 9.
Abstract Link:	http://www.medifocus.com/abstracts.php?gid=RH011&ID=19671451

108.

Assessment of salivary gland function in Sjogren's syndrome: the role of salivary gland scintigraphy.

Authors:	Vinagre F; Santos MJ; Prata A; da Silva JC; Santos AI
Institution:	Rheumatology Department, Hospital Garcia de Orta, Almada, Portugal. filipevinagre@netcabo.pt
Journal:	Autoimmun Rev. 2009 Jul;8(8):672-6. Epub 2009 Feb 24.
Abstract Link:	http://www.medifocus.com/abstracts.php?gid=RH011&ID=19245858

Go to http://www.medifocus.com/links/RH011/0112 for direct online access to the above Abstract Links.

109.

Atrophic change of tongue papilla in 44 patients with Sjogren syndrome.

Authors:	Yamamoto K; Kurihara M; Matsusue Y; Komatsu Y; Tsuyuki M; Fujimoto T; Nakamura S; Kirita T
Institution:	Department of Oral and Maxillofacial Surgery, Nara Medical University, Nara, Japan. kazuyama@naramed-u.ac.jp
Journal:	Oral Surg Oral Med Oral Pathol Oral Radiol Endod. 2009 Jun;107(6):801-5.
Abstract Link:	http://www.medifocus.com/abstracts.php?gid=RH011&ID=19464655

110.

Autoimmune thyroid diseases in a large group of Hungarian patients with primary Sjogren's syndrome.

Authors:	Zeher M; Horvath IF; Szanto A; Szodoray P
Institution:	Division of Clinical Immunology, Medical and Health Science Center, University of Debrecen, Debrecen, Hungary.
Journal:	Thyroid. 2009 Jan;19(1):39-45.
Abstract Link:	http://www.medifocus.com/abstracts.php?gid=RH011&ID=19119981

111.

Association between IFN-alpha and primary Sjogren's syndrome.

Authors:	Zheng L; Zhang Z; Yu C; Tu L; Zhong L; Yang C
Institution:	Department of Oral and Maxillofacial Surgery, Ninth People's Hospital, School of Stomatology, Shanghai Jiao Tong University School of Medicine, Shanghai, China.
Journal:	Oral Surg Oral Med Oral Pathol Oral Radiol Endod. 2009 Jan;107(1):e12-8.
Abstract Link:	http://www.medifocus.com/abstracts.php?gid=RH011&ID=19101478

Go to http://www.medifocus.com/links/RH011/0112 for direct online access to the above Abstract Links.

112.

Safety and usefulness of minor salivary gland biopsy: retrospective analysis of 502 procedures performed at a single center.

Authors:	Caporali R; Bonacci E; Epis O; Bobbio-Pallavicini F; Morbini P; Montecucco C
Institution:	Department of Rheumatology, University of Pavia, IRCCS San Matteo Foundation, Pavia, Italy. caporali@smatteo.pv.it
Journal:	Arthritis Rheum. 2008 May 15;59(5):714-20.
Abstract Link:	http://www.medifocus.com/abstracts.php?gid=RH011&ID=18438907

113.

Fatigue and blood pressure in primary Sjogren's syndrome.

Authors:	d'Elia HF; Rehnberg E; Kvist G; Ericsson A; Konttinen Y; Mannerkorpi K
Institution:	Department of Rheumatology and Inflammation Research, Sahlgrenska Academy, Goteborg University, Sweden. helena.forsblad@vgregion.se
Journal:	Scand J Rheumatol. 2008 Jul-Aug;37(4):284-92.
Abstract Link:	http://www.medifocus.com/abstracts.php?gid=RH011&ID=18612929

114.

Incidence of thromboembolic events in patients with primary Sjogren's syndrome.

Authors:	Haga HJ; Jacobsen EM; Peen E
Institution:	Aalborg University, Esbjerg, Denmark. hjh@reumaklinikdenmark.dk
Journal:	Scand J Rheumatol. 2008 Mar-Apr;37(2):127-9.
Abstract Link:	http://www.medifocus.com/abstracts.php?gid=RH011&ID=18415770

Go to http://www.medifocus.com/links/RH011/0112 for direct online access to the above Abstract Links.

115.

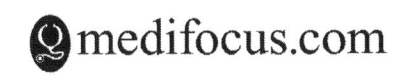

Prevalence and longterm course of primary biliary cirrhosis in primary Sjogren's syndrome.

Authors:	Hatzis GS; Fragoulis GE; Karatzaferis A; Delladetsima I; Barbatis C; Moutsopoulos HM
Institution:	Department of Pathophysiology, National University of Athens Medical School, and Department of Pathology, Red Cross Hospital, Athens, Greece.
Journal:	J Rheumatol. 2008 Oct;35(10):2012-6. Epub 2008 Aug 15.
Abstract Link:	http://www.medifocus.com/abstracts.php?gid=RH011&ID=18709690

116.

Primary Sjogren's syndrome in men: clinical and immunological characteristic based on a large cohort of Hungarian patients.

Authors:	Horvath IF; Szodoray P; Zeher M
Institution:	Division of Clinical Immunology, 3rd Department of Medicine, Medical and Health Science Center, University of Debrecen, Debrecen, Hungary. fanny.horvath@gmail.com
Journal:	Clin Rheumatol. 2008 Dec;27(12):1479-83. Epub 2008 Jun 14.
Abstract Link:	http://www.medifocus.com/abstracts.php?gid=RH011&ID=18553114

117.

Sjogren's syndrome - not just Sicca: renal involvement in Sjogren's syndrome.

Authors:	Kaufman I; Schwartz D; Caspi D; Paran D
Institution:	Department of Rheumatology, Tel Aviv Sourasky Medical Centre, Tel Aviv University, Tel Aviv, Israel. LKaufman@013.net
Journal:	Scand J Rheumatol. 2008 May-Jun;37(3):213-8.
Abstract Link:	http://www.medifocus.com/abstracts.php?gid=RH011&ID=18465457

Go to http://www.medifocus.com/links/RH011/0112 for direct online access to the above Abstract Links.

118.

Sjogren's syndrome sufferers have increased oral yeast levels despite regular dental care.

Authors:	Leung KC; McMillan AS; Cheung BP; Leung WK
Institution:	Oral Rehabilitation, Faculty of Dentistry, The University of Hong Kong, Hong Kong, China.
Journal:	Oral Dis. 2008 Mar;14(2):163-73.
Abstract Link:	http://www.medifocus.com/abstracts.php?gid=RH011&ID=18302677

119.

Interstitial lung disease and Sjogren's syndrome in primary biliary cirrhosis: a causal or casual association?

Authors:	Liu B; Zhang FC; Zhang ZL; Zhang W; Gao LX
Institution:	Department of Rheumatology, Peking Union Medical College Hospital, Chinese Academy of Medical Science, No. 1 Shuai Fu Yuan, Dongcheng District, Beijing, 100730, China.
Journal:	Clin Rheumatol. 2008 Oct;27(10):1299-306. Epub 2008 May 30.
Abstract Link:	http://www.medifocus.com/abstracts.php?gid=RH011&ID=18512115

120.

Autonomic nervous symptoms in primary Sjogren's syndrome.

Authors:	Mandl T; Granberg V; Apelqvist J; Wollmer P; Manthorpe R; Jacobsson LT
Institution:	Department of Rheumatology, Ing 25 plan 2, Malmo University Hospital, S-205 02 Malmo, Sweden. thomas.mandl@med.lu.se
Journal:	Rheumatology (Oxford). 2008 Jun;47(6):914-9. Epub 2008 Apr 14.
Abstract Link:	http://www.medifocus.com/abstracts.php?gid=RH011&ID=18411214

Go to http://www.medifocus.com/links/RH011/0112 for direct online access to the above Abstract Links.

121.

Sjogren's syndrome and localized nodular cutaneous amyloidosis: coincidence or a distinct clinical entity?

Authors:	Meijer JM; Schonland SO; Palladini G; Merlini G; Hegenbart U; Ciocca O; Perfetti V; Leijsma MK; Bootsma H; Hazenberg BP
Institution:	University of Groningen, Groningen, The Netherlands.
Journal:	Arthritis Rheum. 2008 Jul;58(7):1992-9.
Abstract Link:	http://www.medifocus.com/abstracts.php?gid=RH011&ID=18576343

122.

Prevalence, severity, and predictors of fatigue in subjects with primary Sjogren's syndrome.

Authors:	Segal B; Thomas W; Rogers T; Leon JM; Hughes P; Patel D; Patel K; Novitzke J; Rohrer M; Gopalakrishnan R; Myers S; Nazmul-Hossain A; Emamian E; Huang A; Rhodus N; Moser K
Institution:	University of Minnesota, Minneapolis, MN, USA. segal017@umn.edu
Journal:	Arthritis Rheum. 2008 Dec 15;59(12):1780-7.
Abstract Link:	http://www.medifocus.com/abstracts.php?gid=RH011&ID=19035421

123.

Salivary dysfunction and quality of life in Sjogren syndrome: a critical oral-systemic connection.

Authors:	Stewart CM; Berg KM; Cha S; Reeves WH
Institution:	Department of Oral and Maxillofacial Surgery and Diagnostic Sciences, University of Florida, Gainesville 32610, USA. cstewart@dental.ufl.edu
Journal:	J Am Dent Assoc. 2008 Mar;139(3):291-9; quiz 358-9.
Abstract Link:	http://www.medifocus.com/abstracts.php?gid=RH011&ID=18310733

Go to http://www.medifocus.com/links/RH011/0112 for direct online access to the above Abstract Links.

124.

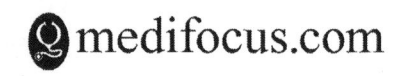

Labial salivary gland biopsies in Sjogren's syndrome: still the gold standard?

Authors:	Stewart CM; Bhattacharyya I; Berg K; Cohen DM; Orlando C; Drew P; Islam NM; Ojha J; Reeves W
Institution:	Department of Oral and Maxillofacial Surgery and Diagnostic Sciences, University of Florida College of Dentistry, Gainesville, FL 32610, USA. cstewart@dental.ufl.edu
Journal:	Oral Surg Oral Med Oral Pathol Oral Radiol Endod. 2008 Sep;106(3):392-402. Epub 2008 Jul 7.
Abstract Link:	http://www.medifocus.com/abstracts.php?gid=RH011&ID=18602295

125.

Alterations in corneal sensitivity and nerve morphology in patients with primary Sjogren's syndrome.

Authors:	Tuisku IS; Konttinen YT; Konttinen LM; Tervo TM
Institution:	Helsinki University Eye Hospital, Helsinki, Finland. ilpo.tuisku@hus.fi
Journal:	Exp Eye Res. 2008 Jun;86(6):879-85. Epub 2008 Mar 12.
Abstract Link:	http://www.medifocus.com/abstracts.php?gid=RH011&ID=18436208

Go to http://www.medifocus.com/links/RH011/0112 for direct online access to the above Abstract Links.

Drug Therapy Articles

126.

Efficacy and safety of orally administered pilocarpine hydrochloride for patients with juvenile-onset Sjogren's syndrome.

Authors:	Tomiita M; Takei S; Kuwada N; Nonaka Y; Saito K; Shimojo N; Kohno Y
Institution:	Department of Pediatrics, Graduate School of Medicine, Chiba University, 1-8-1 Inohana, Chuo-ku, Chiba, Chiba 260-8670, Japan. tomiita@faculty.chiba-u.jp
Journal:	Mod Rheumatol. 2010 Oct;20(5):486-90. Epub 2010 Jun 3.
Abstract Link:	http://www.medifocus.com/abstracts.php?gid=RH011&ID=20517630

127.

Rituximab therapy in primary Sjogren's syndrome.

Authors:	Alcantara C; Gomes MJ; Ferreira C
Institution:	Servico Medicina I, Hospital Santa Maria, Lisbon, Portugal. cristina.alcantara@hsm.min-saude.pt
Journal:	Ann N Y Acad Sci. 2009 Sep;1173:701-5.
Abstract Link:	http://www.medifocus.com/abstracts.php?gid=RH011&ID=19758218

128.

High-frequency Topical Cyclosporine 0.05% in the Treatment of Severe Dry Eye Refractory to Twice-daily Regimen.

Authors:	Dastjerdi MH; Hamrah P; Dana R
Institution:	From the Cornea and Refractive Surgery Service, Massachusetts Eye & Ear Infirmary, Department of Ophthalmology, Harvard Medical School, Boston, MA.
Journal:	Cornea. 2009 Oct 5.
Abstract Link:	http://www.medifocus.com/abstracts.php?gid=RH011&ID=19770713

Go to http://www.medifocus.com/links/RH011/0112 for direct online access to the above Abstract Links.

129.

Sjogren's syndrome patients presenting with hypergammaglobulinemia are relatively unresponsive to cevimeline treatment.

Authors:	Komai K; Shiozawa K; Tanaka Y; Yoshihara R; Tanaka C; Sakai H; Yamane T; Murata M; Tsumiyama K; Hashiramoto A; Shiozawa S
Institution:	Division of Rheumatology, Department of Medicine and Biophysics, Kobe University Graduate School of Medicine and Health Sciences, 7-10-2 Tomogaoka, Suma-ku, Kobe, 654-0142, Japan.
Journal:	Mod Rheumatol. 2009;19(4):416-9. Epub 2009 May 19.
Abstract Link:	http://www.medifocus.com/abstracts.php?gid=RH011&ID=19452244

130.

Treatment of primary Sjogren syndrome with rituximab: extended follow-up, safety and efficacy of retreatment.

Authors:	Meijer JM; Pijpe J; Vissink A; Kallenberg CG; Bootsma H
Journal:	Ann Rheum Dis. 2009 Feb;68(2):284-5.
Abstract Link:	**ABSTRACT NOT AVAILABLE**

131.

Usefulness of initial histological features for stratifying Sjogren's syndrome responders to mizoribine therapy.

Authors:	Nakayamada S; Fujimoto T; Nonomura A; Saito K; Nakamura S; Tanaka Y
Institution:	First Department of Internal Medicine, University of Occupational and Environmental Health, School of Medicine, 1-1 Iseigaoka, Yahatanishi-ku, Kitakyushu 807-8555, Japan.
Journal:	Rheumatology (Oxford). 2009 Oct;48(10):1279-82. Epub 2009 Aug 11.
Abstract Link:	http://www.medifocus.com/abstracts.php?gid=RH011&ID=19671696

Go to http://www.medifocus.com/links/RH011/0112 for direct online access to the above Abstract Links.

132.

Treatment of sicca symptoms with hydroxychloroquine in patients with Sjogren's syndrome.

Authors:	Rihl M; Ulbricht K; Schmidt RE; Witte T
Institution:	Clinic for Immunology and Rheumatology, Hannover Medical School, Hannover, Germany. rihl.markus@mh-hannover.de
Journal:	Rheumatology (Oxford). 2009 Jul;48(7):796-9. Epub 2009 May 11.
Abstract Link:	http://www.medifocus.com/abstracts.php?gid=RH011&ID=19433433

133.

Efficacy and safety of rebamipide for the treatment of dry mouth symptoms in patients with Sjogren's syndrome: a double-blind placebo-controlled multicenter trial.

Authors:	Sugai S; Takahashi H; Ohta S; Nishinarita M; Takei M; Sawada S; Yamaji K; Oka H; Umehara H; Koni I; Sugiyama E; Nishiyama S; Kawakami A
Institution:	Kanazawa Medical University, Ishikawa, Japan, sussugai@helen.ocn.ne.jp.
Journal:	Mod Rheumatol. 2009;19(2):114-24. Epub 2008 Dec 17.
Abstract Link:	http://www.medifocus.com/abstracts.php?gid=RH011&ID=19089532

134.

Effect of Pilocarpine on impaired salivary secretion in patients with Sjogren's syndrome.

Authors:	Jorkjend L; Bergenholtz A; Johansson AK; Johansson A
Institution:	Section of Dental Pharmacology and Pharmacotherapy, University of Oslo, Norway.
Journal:	Swed Dent J. 2008;32(2):49-56.
Abstract Link:	http://www.medifocus.com/abstracts.php?gid=RH011&ID=18700333

Go to http://www.medifocus.com/links/RH011/0112 for direct online access to the above Abstract Links.

Clinical Trials Articles

135.

Clinical features of Sjogren's syndrome in patients with multiple sclerosis.

Authors:	Annunziata P; De Santi L; Di Rezze S; Millefiorini E; Capello E; Mancardi G; De Riz M; Scarpini E; Vecchio R; Patti F
Institution:	Department of Neurological, Neurosurgical and Behavioural Sciences, University of Siena, Siena, Italy. annunziata@unisi.it
Journal:	Acta Neurol Scand. 2011 Aug;124(2):109-14. doi: 10.1111/j.1600-0404.2010.01428.x. Epub 2010 Aug 31.
Abstract Link:	http://www.medifocus.com/abstracts.php?gid=RH011&ID=20809902

136.

Effects of rituximab therapy on quality of life in patients with primary Sjogren's syndrome.

Authors:	Devauchelle-Pensec V; Morvan J; Rat AC; Jousse-Joulin S; Pennec Y; Pers JO; Jamin C; Renaudineau Y; Quintin-Roue I; Cochener B; Youinou P; Saraux A
Institution:	Rheumatology Unit, CHU Brest, France. valerie.devauchelle-pensec@chu-brest.fr
Journal:	Clin Exp Rheumatol. 2011 Jan-Feb;29(1):6-12. Epub 2011 Feb 23.
Abstract Link:	http://www.medifocus.com/abstracts.php?gid=RH011&ID=21345287

137.

Experience of intravenous immunoglobulin therapy in neuropathy associated with primary Sjogren's syndrome: a national multicentric retrospective study.

Authors:	Rist S; Sellam J; Hachulla E; Sordet C; Puechal X; Hatron PY; Benhamou CL; Sibilia J; Mariette X
Institution:	Hopital de la Source, Orleans, France.
Journal:	Arthritis Care Res (Hoboken). 2011 Sep;63(9):1339-44. doi: 10.1002/acr.20495.
Abstract Link:	http://www.medifocus.com/abstracts.php?gid=RH011&ID=21584943

Go to http://www.medifocus.com/links/RH011/0112 for direct online access to the above Abstract Links.

138.

Efficacy and safety of an intraoral electrostimulation device for xerostomia relief: a multicenter, randomized trial.

Authors:	Strietzel FP; Lafaurie GI; Mendoza GR; Alajbeg I; Pejda S; Vuletic L; Mantilla R; Falcao DP; Leal SC; Bezerra AC; Tran SD; Menard HA; Kimoto S; Pan S; Martin-Granizo RA; Lozano ML; Zunt SL; Krushinski CA; Melilli D; Campisi G; Paderni C; Dolce S; Yepes JF; Lindh L; Koray M; Mumcu G; Elad S; Zeevi I; Barrios BC; Lopez Sanchez RM; Beiski BZ; Wolff A; Konttinen YT; Ze
Institution:	Charite Universitatsmedizin Berlin, Berlin, Germany.
Journal:	Arthritis Rheum. 2011 Jan;63(1):180-90. doi: 10.1002/art.27766.
Abstract Link:	http://www.medifocus.com/abstracts.php?gid=RH011&ID=20882668

139.

Effectiveness of rituximab treatment in primary Sjogren's syndrome: a randomized, double-blind, placebo-controlled trial.

Authors:	Meijer JM; Meiners PM; Vissink A; Spijkervet FK; Abdulahad W; Kamminga N; Brouwer E; Kallenberg CG; Bootsma H
Institution:	University Medical Center Groningen, University of Groningen, 9700 RB Groningen, The Netherlands.
Journal:	Arthritis Rheum. 2010 Apr;62(4):960-8.
Abstract Link:	http://www.medifocus.com/abstracts.php?gid=RH011&ID=20131246

140.

Accurate detection of changes in disease activity in primary Sjogren's syndrome by the European League Against Rheumatism Sjogren's Syndrome Disease Activity Index.

Authors:	Seror R; Mariette X; Bowman S; Baron G; Gottenberg JE; Boostma H; Theander E; Tzioufas A; Vitali C; Ravaud P
Institution:	Department of Epidemiology, Biostatistics, and Clinical Research, Hopital Bichat, INSERM U738, 46 rue Henri Huchard, Paris, France. raphaele.se@gmail.com
Journal:	Arthritis Care Res (Hoboken). 2010 Apr;62(4):551-8.
Abstract Link:	http://www.medifocus.com/abstracts.php?gid=RH011&ID=20391511

Go to http://www.medifocus.com/links/RH011/0112 for direct online access to the above Abstract Links.

141.

Dehydroepiandrosterone (DHEA) substitution treatment for severe fatigue in DHEA-deficient patients with primary Sjogren's syndrome.

Authors:	Virkki LM; Porola P; Forsblad-d'Elia H; Valtysdottir S; Solovieva SA; Konttinen YT
Institution:	Helsinki University Central Hospital, Helsinki, Finland.
Journal:	Arthritis Care Res (Hoboken). 2010 Jan 15;62(1):118-24.
Abstract Link:	http://www.medifocus.com/abstracts.php?gid=RH011&ID=20191499

142.

A simplified quantitative method for assessing keratoconjunctivitis sicca from the Sjogren's Syndrome International Registry.

Authors:	Whitcher JP; Shiboski CH; Shiboski SC; Heidenreich AM; Kitagawa K; Zhang S; Hamann S; Larkin G; McNamara NA; Greenspan JS; Daniels TE
Institution:	Department of Ophthalmology, University of California, San Francisco, San Francisco, California 94143-0422, USA.
Journal:	Am J Ophthalmol. 2010 Mar;149(3):405-15. Epub 2009 Dec 29.
Abstract Link:	http://www.medifocus.com/abstracts.php?gid=RH011&ID=20035924

143.

Diagnostic value of salivary gland ultrasonographic scoring system in primary Sjogren's syndrome: a comparison with scintigraphy and biopsy.

Authors:	Milic VD; Petrovic RR; Boricic IV; Marinkovic-Eric J; Radunovic GL; Jeremic PD; Pejnovic NN; Damjanov NS
Institution:	Institute of Rheumatology, Pathology, Social Medicine and Informatics, and Otorhinolaryngology, School of Medicine, University of Belgrade, 11000 Belgrade, Serbia. veramilic@ptt.rs
Journal:	J Rheumatol. 2009 Jul;36(7):1495-500. Epub 2009 Jun 1.
Abstract Link:	http://www.medifocus.com/abstracts.php?gid=RH011&ID=19487274

Go to http://www.medifocus.com/links/RH011/0112 for direct online access to the above Abstract Links.

144.

Clinical and histologic evidence of salivary gland restoration supports the efficacy of rituximab treatment in Sjogren's syndrome.

Authors:	Pijpe J; Meijer JM; Bootsma H; van der Wal JE; Spijkervet FK; Kallenberg CG; Vissink A; Ihrler S
Institution:	University of Groningen, Groningen, The Netherlands.
Journal:	Arthritis Rheum. 2009 Nov;60(11):3251-6.
Abstract Link:	http://www.medifocus.com/abstracts.php?gid=RH011&ID=19877054

145.

Systemic autoimmune diseases in patients with hepatitis C virus infection: characterization of 1020 cases (The HISPAMEC Registry).

Authors:	Ramos-Casals M; Munoz S; Medina F; Jara LJ; Rosas J; Calvo-Alen J; Brito-Zeron P; Forns X; Sanchez-Tapias JM
Institution:	Laboratory of Autoimmune Diseases Josep Font, Department of Autoimmune Diseases, Institut d'Investigacions Biomediques August Pi i Sunyer (IDIBAPS), Hospital Clinic, 08036-Barcelona, Spain. mramos@clinic.ub.es
Journal:	J Rheumatol. 2009 Jul;36(7):1442-8. Epub 2009 Apr 15.
Abstract Link:	http://www.medifocus.com/abstracts.php?gid=RH011&ID=19369460

146.

Reduction of fatigue in Sjogren syndrome with rituximab: results of a randomised, double-blind, placebo-controlled pilot study.

Authors:	Dass S; Bowman SJ; Vital EM; Ikeda K; Pease CT; Hamburger J; Richards A; Rauz S; Emery P
Institution:	Academic Unit of Musculoskeletal Disease, University of Leeds, Leeds, UK.
Journal:	Ann Rheum Dis. 2008 Nov;67(11):1541-4. Epub 2008 Feb 14.
Abstract Link:	http://www.medifocus.com/abstracts.php?gid=RH011&ID=18276741

Go to http://www.medifocus.com/links/RH011/0112 for direct online access to the above Abstract Links.

147.

Oral involvement in primary Sjogren syndrome.

Authors:	Fox PC; Bowman SJ; Segal B; Vivino FB; Murukutla N; Choueiri K; Ogale S; McLean L
Institution:	PC Fox Consulting, Via Monterione, Spello, Italy. pcfox@comcast.net
Journal:	J Am Dent Assoc. 2008 Dec;139(12):1592-601.
Abstract Link:	http://www.medifocus.com/abstracts.php?gid=RH011&ID=19047665

148.

Primary Sjogren's syndrome in men.

Authors:	Gondran G; Fauchais A; Lambert M; Ly K; Launay D; Queyrel V; Benazahari H; Liozon E; Loustaud-Ratti V; Hachulla E; Jauberteau M; Hatron P; Vidal E
Institution:	Internal Medicine Department, Limoges University Hospital, France.
Journal:	Scand J Rheumatol. 2008 Jul-Aug;37(4):300-5.
Abstract Link:	http://www.medifocus.com/abstracts.php?gid=RH011&ID=18612931

149.

Effect of the H2 receptor antagonist nizatidine on xerostomia in patients with primary Sjogren's syndrome.

Authors:	Kasama T; Shiozawa F; Isozaki T; Matsunawa M; Wakabayashi K; Odai T; Yajima N; Miwa Y; Negishi M; Ide H
Institution:	Division of Rheumatology, Department of Internal Medicine, Showa University School of Medicine, 1-5-8 Hatanodai, Shinagawa-ku, Tokyo, 142-8666, Japan. tkasama@med.showa-u.ac.jp
Journal:	Mod Rheumatol. 2008;18(5):455-9. Epub 2008 May 14.
Abstract Link:	http://www.medifocus.com/abstracts.php?gid=RH011&ID=18478182

Go to http://www.medifocus.com/links/RH011/0112 for direct online access to the above Abstract Links.

150.

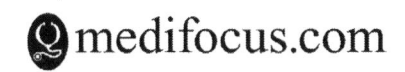

The efficacy of cevimeline hydrochloride in the treatment of xerostomia in Sjogren's syndrome in southern Chinese patients: a randomised double-blind, placebo-controlled crossover study.

Authors: Leung KC; McMillan AS; Wong MC; Leung WK; Mok MY; Lau CS
Institution: Oral Rehabilitation, Faculty of Dentistry, The University of Hong Kong, Hong Kong, China.
Journal: Clin Rheumatol. 2008 Apr;27(4):429-36. Epub 2007 Sep 26.
Abstract Link: http://www.medifocus.com/abstracts.php?gid=RH011&ID=17899308

NOTES

Use this page for taking notes as you review your Guidebook

4 - Centers of Research

This section of your *MediFocus Guidebook* is a unique directory of doctors, researchers, medical centers, and research institutions with specialized research interest, and in many cases, clinical expertise in the management of this specific medical condition. The *Centers of Research* directory is a valuable resource for quickly identifying and locating leading medical authorities and medical institutions within the United States and other countries that are considered to be at the forefront in clinical research and treatment of this disorder.

Use the *Centers of Research* directory to contact, consult, or network with leading experts in the field and to locate a hospital or medical center that can help you.

The following information is provided in the *Centers of Research* directory:

- **Geographic Location**

    - United States: the information is divided by individual states listed in alphabetical order. Not all states may be included.

    - Other Countries: information is presented for select countries worldwide listed in alphabetical order. Not all countries may be included.

- **Names of Authors**

    - Select names of individual authors (doctors, researchers, or other health-care professionals) with specialized research interest, and in many cases, clinical expertise in the management of this specific medical condition, who have recently published articles in leading medical journals about the condition.

    - E-mail addresses for individual authors, if listed on their specific publications, is also provided.

- **Institutional Affiliations**

    - Next to each individual author's name is their **institutional affiliation** (hospital, medical center, or research institution) where the study was conducted as listed in their publication(s).

- In many cases, information about the specific **department** within the medical institution where the individual author was located at the time the study was conducted is also provided.

Centers of Research

United States

CA - California

Name of Author	Institutional Affiliation
Daniels TE	Department of Ophthalmology, University of California, San Francisco, San Francisco, California 94143-0422, USA.
Nazmul-Hossain AN	Dental Research Institute, University of California, Los Angeles, USA.
Rhodus NL	Dental Research Institute, University of California, Los Angeles, USA.
Whitcher JP	Department of Ophthalmology, University of California, San Francisco, San Francisco, California 94143-0422, USA.
Wu AJ	Sjogren's Syndrome Clinic, University of California, San Francisco, 513 Parnassus Avenue, Room C646, CA 94143, USA. ava.wu@ucsf.edu

CO - Colorado

Name of Author	Institutional Affiliation
Brown KK	Autoimmune and Interstitial Lung Disease Program, Department of Medicine, National Jewish Health, 1400 Jackson St, Denver, CO 80206, USA. fischera@njhealth.org
Fischer A	Autoimmune and Interstitial Lung Disease Program, Department of Medicine, National Jewish Health, 1400 Jackson St, Denver, CO 80206, USA. fischera@njhealth.org

CT - Connecticut

Name of Author	Institutional Affiliation
Parke AL	Division of Rheumatology, Saint Francis Hospital and Medical Center, 114 Woodland Street, Hartford, CT 06105-1208, USA.

FL - Florida

Name of Author	Institutional Affiliation
Reeves W	Department of Oral and Maxillofacial Surgery and Diagnostic Sciences, University of Florida College of Dentistry, Gainesville, FL 32610, USA. cstewart@dental.ufl.edu
Reeves WH	Department of Oral and Maxillofacial Surgery and Diagnostic Sciences, University of Florida, Gainesville 32610, USA. cstewart@dental.ufl.edu
Stewart CM	Department of Oral and Maxillofacial Surgery and Diagnostic Sciences, University of Florida, Gainesville 32610, USA. cstewart@dental.ufl.edu

IL - Illinois

Name of Author	Institutional Affiliation
Bamba R	Pritzker School of Medicine, University of Chicago, Chicago, Illinois, U.S.A.
Blair EA	Pritzker School of Medicine, University of Chicago, Chicago, Illinois, U.S.A.
Logemann JA	Department of Communication Sciences and Disorders, Northwestern University, Evanston, IL, 60208-3570, USA, nicoleroguspulia@gmail.com.
Rogus-Pulia NM	Department of Communication Sciences and Disorders, Northwestern University, Evanston, IL, 60208-3570, USA, nicoleroguspulia@gmail.com.

KY - Kentucky

Name of Author	Institutional Affiliation
Foulks GN	Department of Ophthalmology and Visual Sciences, University of Louisville School of Medicine, 301 East Muhammad Ali Boulevard, Louisville, KY 40202, USA. gnfoul01@louisville.edu

MA - Massachussetts

Name of Author	Institutional Affiliation
Dana R	From the Cornea and Refractive Surgery Service, Massachusetts Eye & Ear Infirmary, Department of Ophthalmology, Harvard Medical School, Boston, MA.
Dastjerdi MH	From the Cornea and Refractive Surgery Service, Massachusetts Eye & Ear Infirmary, Department of Ophthalmology, Harvard Medical School, Boston, MA.
Davis M	Massachusetts General Hospital, Harvard Medical School, Charlestown, MA 02129, USA. faustman@helix.mgh.harvard.edu
Faustman DL	Massachusetts General Hospital, Harvard Medical School, Charlestown, MA 02129, USA. faustman@helix.mgh.harvard.edu
Papas AS	Division of Oral Medicine and Dental Research, Tufts University School of Dental Medicine, Boston, Massachusetts, USA. periodok@yahoo.com
Singh M	Division of Oral Medicine and Dental Research, Tufts University School of Dental Medicine, Boston, Massachusetts, USA. periodok@yahoo.com

MD - Maryland

Name of Author	Institutional Affiliation
Akpek EK	The Wilmer Eye Institute, The Johns Hopkins University School of Medicine, Baltimore, MD, USA. esakpek@jhmi.edu
Baer AN	Division of Rheumatology, Good Samaritan Hospital, Russell Morgan Building, Suite 508, 5601 Loch Raven Blvd., Baltimore, MD 21239, USA. alanbaer@jhmi.edu
Birnbaum J	Department of Neurology, The Johns Hopkins Jerome Greene Sjogren's Center, Baltimore, MD, USA. jbirnba2@jhmi.edu
Illei GG	Molecular Physiology and Therapeutics Branch, National Institute of Dental and Craniofacial Research, National Institutes of Health, DHHS, Bethesda, MD, USA.
Kruszka P	U.S. Coast Guard Yard, Baltimore, Maryland, USA. paul_kruszka@hotmail.com
McDonnell PJ	The Wilmer Eye Institute, The Johns Hopkins University School of Medicine, Baltimore, MD, USA. esakpek@jhmi.edu
Nikolov NP	Sjogren's Syndrome Clinic, National Institute of Dental and Craniofacial Research (NIDCR), Molecular Physiology and Therapeutics Branch, National Institutes of Health (NIH), Bethesda, Maryland 20892, USA.
O'Brian RJ	U.S. Coast Guard Yard, Baltimore, Maryland, USA. paul_kruszka@hotmail.com
Ostrovsky A	Ocular Surface Diseases and Dry Eye Clinic, Division of Cornea, Wilmer Eye Institute, The Johns Hopkins University School of Medicine, Baltimore, MD, USA. esakpek@jhmi.edu
Petri M	Division of Rheumatology, Good Samaritan Hospital, Russell Morgan Building, Suite 508, 5601 Loch Raven Blvd., Baltimore, MD 21239, USA. alanbaer@jhmi.edu
Roescher N	Molecular Physiology and Therapeutics Branch, National Institute of Dental and Craniofacial Research, National Institutes of Health, DHHS, Bethesda, MD, USA.

MN - Minnesota

Name of Author	Institutional Affiliation
Gabriel SE	Department of Health Sciences Research, Mayo Foundation, Rochester, MN 55905, USA. gabriel.sherine@mayo.edu
Hogan MC	Department of Internal Medicine, Mayo Clinic, Rochester, Minnesota 55905, USA.
Maripuri S	Department of Internal Medicine, Mayo Clinic, Rochester, Minnesota 55905, USA.
McLean L	Associate Professor, Division of Rheumatic and Autoimmune Diseases, Department of Medicine, University of Minnesota, USA. segal017@umn.edu
Michaud K	Department of Health Sciences Research, Mayo Foundation, Rochester, MN 55905, USA. gabriel.sherine@mayo.edu
Moser K	University of Minnesota, Minneapolis, MN, USA. segal017@umn.edu
Segal B	University of Minnesota, Minneapolis, MN, USA. segal017@umn.edu
Walk D	Division of Rheumatic and Autoimmune Disorders, University of Minnesota Medical School, MMC 108, 420 Delaware SE, Minneapolis, MN 55455, USA. segal017@umn.edu

NY - New York

Name of Author	Institutional Affiliation
Carsons SE	SUNY at Stony Brook School of Medicine, Stony Brook, NY, USA. Scarsons@winthrop.org
Coca A	Division of Allergy, Immunology and Rheumatology, University of Rochester, Rochester, New York 14642, USA.
Sanz I	Division of Allergy, Immunology and Rheumatology, University of Rochester, Rochester, New York 14642, USA.

OH - Ohio

Name of Author	Institutional Affiliation
Awad A	Neurological Institute, University Hospitals Case Medical Center, Case Western Reserve University, Cleveland, Ohio 44104, USA. ameraldo@gmail.com
Katirji B	Neurological Institute, University Hospitals Case Medical Center, Case Western Reserve University, Cleveland, Ohio 44104, USA. ameraldo@gmail.com
Lowe R	Division of Pediatric Infectious Diseases and Rheumatology, Rainbow Babies and Children's Hospital, Cleveland, OH 44106, USA. nora.singer@uhhospitals.org
Singer NG	Division of Pediatric Infectious Diseases and Rheumatology, Rainbow Babies and Children's Hospital, Cleveland, OH 44106, USA. nora.singer@uhhospitals.org
Wander AH	Department of Ophthalmology, University of Cincinnati College of Medicine and Academic Health Center, Cincinnati, OH, USA. myersdo@ucphysicians.com

OK - Oklahoma

Name of Author	Institutional Affiliation
Cobb BL	Arthritis and Immunology Program, Oklahoma Medical Research Foundation, 825 NE 13th Street, Oklahoma City, OK 73104, USA.
James JA	Arthritis and Immunology Program, Oklahoma Medical Research Foundation, Oklahoma City, Oklahoma 73104, USA.
Mathews SA	University of Central Oklahoma, Edmond, OK, USA.
Moser KL	Arthritis and Immunology Program, Oklahoma Medical Research Foundation, 825 NE 13th Street, Oklahoma City, OK 73104, USA.
Scofield RH	University of Central Oklahoma, Edmond, OK, USA.
Thanou-Stavraki A	Arthritis and Immunology Program, Oklahoma Medical Research Foundation, Oklahoma City, Oklahoma 73104, USA.

PA - Pennsylvania

Name of Author	Institutional Affiliation
Hermann GA	Penn Presbyterian Medical Center, Penn Sjogren's Syndrome Center, University of Pennsylvania School of Medicine, 51 North 39th Street, 3910 Building, Philadelphia, PA 19104, USA. frederick.vivino@uphs.upenn.edu
Kittridge A	West Penn Allegheny Health System, Department of Medicine , Pittsburg, PA, USA.
Korman NJ	West Penn Allegheny Health System, Department of Medicine , Pittsburg, PA, USA.
Vivino FB	Penn Presbyterian Medical Center, Penn Sjogren's Syndrome Center, University of Pennsylvania School of Medicine, 51 North 39th Street, 3910 Building, Philadelphia, PA 19104, USA. frederick.vivino@uphs.upenn.edu

TX - Texas

Name of Author	Institutional Affiliation
Hall DA	Amarillo College in Amarillo, Texas, USA.
Pullen RL Jr	Amarillo College in Amarillo, Texas, USA.

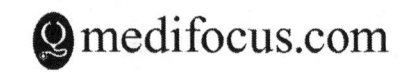

Centers of Research

Other Countries

Brazil

Name of Author	Institutional Affiliation
Antoniazzi RP	Postgraduate Program in Dentistry, Brazilian Lutheran University, Canoas, RS, Brazil. raquelantoniazzi@hotmail.com
Hida RY	Department of Ophthalmology, Hospital das Clinicas of University of Sao Paulo, Brazil.
Holzchuh R	Department of Ophthalmology, Hospital das Clinicas of University of Sao Paulo, Brazil.
Oppermann RV	Postgraduate Program in Dentistry, Brazilian Lutheran University, Canoas, RS, Brazil. raquelantoniazzi@hotmail.com

Canada

Name of Author	Institutional Affiliation
Bell DA	Department of Medicine, Division of Rheumatology, St Joseph's Health Care London and University of Western Ontario, London, Ontario, Canada.
George A	Schulich School of Medicine, University of Western Ontario, London, Ontario, Canada.
Mohammed K	Department of Medicine, Division of Rheumatology, St Joseph's Health Care London and University of Western Ontario, London, Ontario, Canada.
Pope JE	Schulich School of Medicine, University of Western Ontario, London, Ontario, Canada.

China

Name of Author	Institutional Affiliation
Chapin WJ	Department of Ophthalmology, EYE & ENT Hospital of Fudan University, No. 83 Fenyang Road, Shanghai, China.
Gao LX	Department of Rheumatology, Peking Union Medical College Hospital, Chinese Academy of Medical Science, No. 1 Shuai Fu Yuan, Dongcheng District, Beijing, 100730, China.
Lau CS	Oral Rehabilitation, Faculty of Dentistry, The University of Hong Kong, Hong Kong, China.
Leung KC	Oral Rehabilitation, Faculty of Dentistry, The University of Hong Kong, Hong Kong, China.
Li M	Department of Ophthalmology, EYE & ENT Hospital of Fudan University, No. 83 Fenyang Road, Shanghai, China.
Liu B	Department of Rheumatology, Peking Union Medical College Hospital, Chinese Academy of Medical Science, No. 1 Shuai Fu Yuan, Dongcheng District, Beijing, 100730, China.
Shi JH	Department of Pulmonary Medicine, Peking Union Medical College Hospital, Chinese Academy of Medical Science and Peking Union Medical College, Beijing, China.
Xu D	Department of Rheumatology, Peking Union Medical College (PUMC) Hospital, Chinese Academy of Medical Sciences and Peking Union Medical College, Beijing 100730, China.
Yang C	Department of Oral and Maxillofacial Surgery, Ninth People's Hospital, School of Stomatology, Shanghai Jiao Tong University School of Medicine, Shanghai, China.
Zhang F	Department of Rheumatology, Peking Union Medical College (PUMC) Hospital, Chinese Academy of Medical Sciences and Peking Union Medical College, Beijing 100730, China.
Zheng L	Department of Oral and Maxillofacial Surgery, Ninth People's Hospital, School of Stomatology, Shanghai Jiao Tong University School of Medicine, Shanghai, China.

| Zhu YJ | Department of Pulmonary Medicine, Peking Union Medical College Hospital, Chinese Academy of Medical Science and Peking Union Medical College, Beijing, China. |

Czech Republic

Name of Author	Institutional Affiliation
Brunova B	Department of Eye Histochemistry and Pharmacology, Institute of Experimental Medicine, Academy of Sciences of the Czech Republic, Prague, Czech Republic. cejkova@biomed.cas.cz
Cejkova J	Department of Eye Histochemistry and Pharmacology, Institute of Experimental Medicine, Academy of Sciences of the Czech Republic, Prague, Czech Republic. cejkova@biomed.cas.cz

Denmark

Name of Author	Institutional Affiliation
Haga HJ	Aalborg University Esbjerg, Esbjerg, Denmark.
Peen E	Aalborg University Esbjerg, Esbjerg, Denmark.

Finland

Name of Author	Institutional Affiliation
Konttinen YT	Helsinki University Central Hospital, Helsinki, Finland.
Parkkila S	Department of Internal Medicine, Rheumatology Centre, Tampere University Hospital, Tampere, Finland. marja.pertovaara@uta.fi
Pertovaara M	Department of Internal Medicine, Rheumatology Centre, Tampere University Hospital, Tampere, Finland. marja.pertovaara@uta.fi
Tervo TM	Helsinki University Eye Hospital, Helsinki, Finland. ilpo.tuisku@hus.fi

Tuisku IS	Helsinki University Eye Hospital, Helsinki, Finland. ilpo.tuisku@hus.fi
Virkki LM	Helsinki University Central Hospital, Helsinki, Finland.

France

Name of Author	Institutional Affiliation
Borie R	Assistance Publique-Hopitaux de Paris, Hopital Bichat, Service de Pneumologie A, Centre de Competence maladies rares pulmonaires, Paris, France.
Cacoub P	Service de Medecine Interne, AP-HP, Hopital Pitie-Salpetriere, and Universite Pierre et Marie Curie-Paris 6, Paris, France. damien.sene@psl.aphp.fr
Crestani B	Assistance Publique-Hopitaux de Paris, Hopital Bichat, Service de Pneumologie A, Centre de Competence maladies rares pulmonaires, Paris, France.
Devauchelle-Pensec V	Rheumatology Unit, CHU Brest, France. valerie.devauchelle-pensec@chu-brest.fr
Gondran G	Internal Medicine Department, Limoges University Hospital, France.
Gottenberg JE	Hopital Bicetre, Assistance Publique-Hopitaux de Paris, Universite Paris-Sud 11, Institut Pour la Sante et la Recherche Medicale U1012, Le Kremlin Bicetre, France. xavier.mariette@bct.aphp.fr
Mariette X	Hopital de la Source, Orleans, France.
Michel L	Service de Neurologie, Centre Hospitalier Universitaire de Nantes, Hopital Laennec, Nantes Cedex, France. Laure.michel@univ-nantes.fr
Ravaud P	Department of Epidemiology, Biostatistics, and Clinical Research, Hopital Bichat, INSERM U738, 46 rue Henri Huchard, Paris, France. raphaele.se@gmail.com
Rist S	Hopital de la Source, Orleans, France.
Saraux A	EA2216, IFR148, Universite de Bretagne Occidentale, Brest, France; Service de Rhumatologie, Centre Hospitalier Universitaire de Brest, Brest, France.

Sene D	Service de Medecine Interne, AP-HP, Hopital Pitie-Salpetriere, and Universite Pierre et Marie Curie-Paris 6, Paris, France. damien.sene@psl.aphp.fr
Seror R	Department of Epidemiology, Biostatistics, and Clinical Research, Hopital Bichat, INSERM U738, 46 rue Henri Huchard, Paris, France. raphaele.se@gmail.com
Tobon GJ	EA2216, IFR148, Universite de Bretagne Occidentale, Brest, France; Service de Rhumatologie, Centre Hospitalier Universitaire de Brest, Brest, France.
Vidal E	Internal Medicine Department, Limoges University Hospital, France.
Vitali C	Department of Epidemiology, Biostatistics and Clinical Research, Hopital Bichat, INSERM U738, Hopital Bichat, 46 rue Henri Huchard, Paris 75018, France. raphaele.se@gmail.com
Wiertlewski S	Service de Neurologie, Centre Hospitalier Universitaire de Nantes, Hopital Laennec, Nantes Cedex, France. Laure.michel@univ-nantes.fr

Germany

Name of Author	Institutional Affiliation
Aringer M	Division of Rheumatology, Department of Medicine III, University Center Carl Gustav Carus, Technical University of Dresden, Dresden, Germany.
Becker H	Department of Medicine D, University of Muenster, Muenster, Germany. beckerhe@mednet.uni-muenster.de.
Burmester GR	Charite Center 12 and 14, Charite University Hospital & Deutsches Rheuma-Forschungszentrum Berlin, Berlin, Germany. thomas.doerner@charite.de
Dorner T	Charite Center 12 and 14, Charite University Hospital & Deutsches Rheuma-Forschungszentrum Berlin, Berlin, Germany. thomas.doerner@charite.de
Konttinen YT	Charite Universitatsmedizin Berlin, Berlin, Germany.
Rihl M	Clinic for Immunology and Rheumatology, Hannover Medical School, Hannover, Germany. rihl.markus@mh-hannover.de

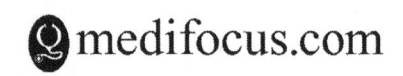

Strietzel FP	Charite Universitatsmedizin Berlin, Berlin, Germany.
Willeke P	Department of Medicine D, University of Muenster, Muenster, Germany. beckerhe@mednet.uni-muenster.de.
Winzer M	Division of Rheumatology, Department of Medicine III, University Center Carl Gustav Carus, Technical University of Dresden, Dresden, Germany.
Witte T	Clinic for Immunology and Rheumatology, Hannover Medical School, Hannover, Germany. rihl.markus@mh-hannover.de

Greece

Name of Author	Institutional Affiliation
Baimpa E	Department of Pathophysiology, Medical School of Athens, National University of Athens, Athens, Greece.
Dalakas MC	Department of Pathophysiology, Medical School, University of Athens, Athens, Greece.
Drosos AA	Department of Psychiatry, Medical School, University of Ioannina, Ioannina, Greece.
Hatzis GS	Department of Pathophysiology, National University of Athens Medical School, and Department of Pathology, Red Cross Hospital, Athens, Greece.
Highland KB	3rd Pulmonary Department, Sismanoglio General Hospital, Athens, Greece.
Hyphantis T	Department of Psychiatry, Medical School, University of Ioannina, Ioannina, Greece.
Karaiskos D	Department of Pathophysiology, School of Medicine, University of Athens, Athens, Greece.
Kokosi M	3rd Pulmonary Department, Sismanoglio General Hospital, Athens, Greece.
Moutsopoulos HM	Department of Pathophysiology, Medical School, National University of Athens, Greece.
Pavlakis PP	Department of Pathophysiology, Medical School, University of Athens, Athens, Greece.

Tzioufas AG	Department of Pathophysiology, School of Medicine, University of Athens, Athens, Greece. agtzi@med.uoa.gr
Voulgarelis M	Department of Pathophysiology, Medical School, National University of Athens, Greece.

Hungary

Name of Author	Institutional Affiliation
Horvath IF	Division of Clinical Immunology, 3rd Department of Medicine, Medical and Health Science Center, University of Debrecen, Debrecen, Hungary. fanny.horvath@gmail.com
Kiss E	Department of Rheumatology, Albert Szent-Gyorgyi Clinical Centre, University of Szeged, Hungary.
Kovacs L	Department of Rheumatology, Albert Szent-Gyorgyi Clinical Centre, University of Szeged, Hungary.
Szodoray P	Division of Clinical Immunology, Medical and Health Science Center, University of Debrecen , Debrecen, Hungary.
Zeher M	Division of Clinical Immunology, Medical and Health Science Center, University of Debrecen , Debrecen, Hungary.

India

Name of Author	Institutional Affiliation
Gupta D	Department of Pulmonary Medicine, Postgraduate Institute of Medical Education and Research (PGIMER), Chandigarh, India. visitsrinivasan@gmail.com
Rajagopala S	Department of Pulmonary Medicine, Postgraduate Institute of Medical Education and Research (PGIMER), Chandigarh, India. visitsrinivasan@gmail.com

Israel

Name of Author	Institutional Affiliation
Kaufman I	Department of Rheumatology, Tel Aviv Sourasky Medical Centre, Tel Aviv University, Tel Aviv, Israel. LKaufman@013.net
Nahlieli O	Department of Oral and Maxillofacial Surgery, Barzilai Medical Center, Ashkelon, Israel.
Paran D	Department of Rheumatology, Tel Aviv Sourasky Medical Centre, Tel Aviv University, Tel Aviv, Israel. LKaufman@013.net
Shacham R	Department of Oral and Maxillofacial Surgery, Barzilai Medical Center, Ashkelon, Israel.

Italy

Name of Author	Institutional Affiliation
Annunziata P	Department of Neurological, Neurosurgical and Behavioural Sciences, University of Siena, Siena, Italy. annunziata@unisi.it
Botsios C	Rheumatology Unit, Department of Clinical and Experimental Medicine, University of Padova, via Giustiniani 2, 35128 Padova, Italy. constantin.botsios@unipd.it
Caporali R	Department of Rheumatology, University of Pavia, IRCCS San Matteo Foundation, Pavia, Italy. caporali@smatteo.pv.it
Di Franco M	Dipartimento di Medicina Interna e Specialita Mediche, Reumatologia, Universita La Sapienza, Rome, Italy. rob.pri@libero.it
Fox PC	PC Fox Consulting, Via Monterione, Spello, Italy. pcfox@comcast.net
McLean L	PC Fox Consulting, Via Monterione, Spello, Italy. pcfox@comcast.net
Montecucco C	Department of Rheumatology, University of Pavia, IRCCS San Matteo Foundation, Pavia, Italy. caporali@smatteo.pv.it

Patti F	Department of Neurological, Neurosurgical and Behavioural Sciences, University of Siena, Siena, Italy. annunziata@unisi.it
Priori R	Dipartimento di Medicina Interna e Specialita Mediche, Reumatologia, Universita La Sapienza, Rome, Italy. rob.pri@libero.it
Punzi L	Rheumatology Unit, Department of Clinical and Experimental Medicine, University of Padova, via Giustiniani 2, 35128 Padova, Italy. constantin.botsios@unipd.it
Vitali C	Department of Internal Medicine and Section of Rheumatology, 'Villamarina' Hospital, Piombino, Italy. c.vitali@yahoo.it

Japan

Name of Author	Institutional Affiliation
Gono T	Institute of Rheumatology, Tokyo Women's Medical University, 10-22 Kawada-cho, Shinjuku-Ku Tokyo 162-0054, Japan.
Goto E	Department of Ophthalmology, School of Dental Medicine, Tsurumi University, 2-1-3 Tsurumi, Yokohama City, Kanagawa, Japan 230-8501. goto-e@tsurumi-u.ac.jp
Ide H	Division of Rheumatology, Department of Internal Medicine, Showa University School of Medicine, 1-5-8 Hatanodai, Shinagawa-ku, Tokyo, 142-8666, Japan. tkasama@med.showa-u.ac.jp
Kasama T	Division of Rheumatology, Department of Internal Medicine, Showa University School of Medicine, 1-5-8 Hatanodai, Shinagawa-ku, Tokyo, 142-8666, Japan. tkasama@med.showa-u.ac.jp
Katayama I	Department of Dermatology, Course of Integrated Medicine, Graduate School of Medicine, Osaka University, 2-2 Yamada-oka, Suita, Osaka, 565-0871, Japan, katayama@derma.med.Osaka-u.ac.jp.

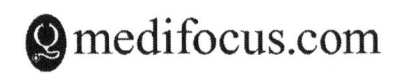

Kawakami A	Kanazawa Medical University, Ishikawa, Japan, sussugai@helen.ocn.ne.jp.
Kirita T	Department of Oral and Maxillofacial Surgery, Nara Medical University, Nara, Japan. kazuyama@naramed-u.ac.jp
Kohno Y	Department of Pediatrics, Graduate School of Medicine, Chiba University, 1-8-1 Inohana, Chuo-ku, Chiba, Chiba 260-8670, Japan. tomiita@faculty.chiba-u.jp
Komai K	Division of Rheumatology, Department of Medicine and Biophysics, Kobe University Graduate School of Medicine and Health Sciences, 7-10-2 Tomogaoka, Suma-ku, Kobe, 654-0142, Japan.
Morozumi S	Department of Neurology, Nagoya University Graduate School of Medicine, Nagoya, Japan.
Murota H	Department of Dermatology, Course of Integrated Medicine, Graduate School of Medicine, Osaka University, 2-2 Yamada-oka, Suita, Osaka, 565-0871, Japan, katayama@derma.med.Osaka-u.ac.jp.
Nakayamada S	First Department of Internal Medicine, University of Occupational and Environmental Health, School of Medicine, 1-1 Iseigaoka, Yahatanishi-ku, Kitakyushu 807-8555, Japan.
Shiozawa S	Division of Rheumatology, Department of Medicine and Biophysics, Kobe University Graduate School of Medicine and Health Sciences, 7-10-2 Tomogaoka, Suma-ku, Kobe, 654-0142, Japan.
Sobue G	Department of Neurology, Nagoya University Graduate School of Medicine, Nagoya, Japan.
Sugai S	Kanazawa Medical University, Ishikawa, Japan, sussugai@helen.ocn.ne.jp.
Tanaka Y	First Department of Internal Medicine, University of Occupational and Environmental Health, School of Medicine, 1-1 Iseigaoka, Yahatanishi-ku, Kitakyushu 807-8555, Japan.
Tomiita M	Department of Pediatrics, Graduate School of Medicine, Chiba University, 1-8-1 Inohana, Chuo-ku, Chiba, Chiba 260-8670, Japan. tomiita@faculty.chiba-u.jp

Tsubota K	Department of Ophthalmology, School of Dental Medicine, Tsurumi University, 2-1-3 Tsurumi, Yokohama City, Kanagawa, Japan 230-8501. goto-e@tsurumi-u.ac.jp
Yamamoto K	Department of Oral and Maxillofacial Surgery, Nara Medical University, Nara, Japan. kazuyama@naramed-u.ac.jp
Yamanaka H	Institute of Rheumatology, Tokyo Women's Medical University, 10-22 Kawada-cho, Shinjuku-Ku Tokyo 162-0054, Japan.

Mexico

Name of Author	Institutional Affiliation
Hernandez-Molina G	Immunology and Rheumatology Department, Instituto Nacional de Ciencias Medicas y Nutricion SZ, Vasco de Quiroga 15. Colonia Seccion XVI, CP 14000, Mexico City, Mexico. gabyhm@yahoo.com
Michel-Peregrina M	Immunology and Rheumatology Department, Instituto Nacional de Ciencias Medicas y Nutricion SZ, Vasco de Quiroga 15. Colonia Seccion XVI, CP 14000, Mexico City, Mexico. gabyhm@yahoo.com
Sanchez-Guerrero J	Department of Immunology and Rheumatology, Ophthalmology Service, and Dental Service, Instituto Nacional de Ciencias Medicas y Nutricion Salvador Zubiran, Mexico City, Mexico.

Netherlands

Name of Author	Institutional Affiliation
Bootsma H	University Medical Center Groningen, University of Groningen, 9700 RB Groningen, The Netherlands.
Geenen R	Department of Clinical and Health Psychology, Utrecht University, Utrecht, The Netherlands. marijnvanoers@gmail.com
Ihrler S	University of Groningen, Groningen, The Netherlands.

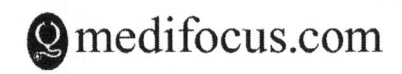

Kelder JC	Department of Rheumatology, St. Antonius Hospital, Nieuwegein, The Netherlands. borg@antoniusziekenhuis.nl
Meijer JM	University of Groningen, Groningen, The Netherlands.
ter Borg EJ	Department of Rheumatology, St. Antonius Hospital, Nieuwegein, The Netherlands. borg@antoniusziekenhuis.nl
van Oers ML	Department of Clinical and Health Psychology, Utrecht University, Utrecht, The Netherlands. marijnvanoers@gmail.com

Norway

Name of Author	Institutional Affiliation
Bolstad AI	Department of Clinical Dentistry - Periodontics, University of Bergen, Bergen, Norway.
Delaleu N	Broegelmann Research Laboratory, The Gade Institute, University of Bergen, Haukelandsveien 28, Bergen 5021, Norway.
Hjelmervik TO	Department of Clinical Dentistry - Periodontics, University of Bergen, Bergen, Norway.
Isaksen K	Department of Internal Medicine, Stavanger University Hospital, Stavanger, Norway. isak@sus.no
Johansson A	Section of Dental Pharmacology and Pharmacotherapy, University of Oslo, Norway.
Jonsson R	Broegelmann Research Laboratory, The Gade Institute, University of Bergen, Haukelandsveien 28, Bergen 5021, Norway.
Jorkjend L	Section of Dental Pharmacology and Pharmacotherapy, University of Oslo, Norway.
Omdal R	Department of Internal Medicine, Stavanger University Hospital, Stavanger, Norway. isak@sus.no

Portugal

Name of Author	Institutional Affiliation
Alcantara C	Servico Medicina I, Hospital Santa Maria, Lisbon, Portugal. cristina.alcantara@hsm.min-saude.pt
Campar A	Santo Antonio Hospital - Centro Hospitalar do Porto, Porto, Portugal.
Ferreira C	Servico Medicina I, Hospital Santa Maria, Lisbon, Portugal. cristina.alcantara@hsm.min-saude.pt
Isenberg DA	Santo Antonio Hospital - Centro Hospitalar do Porto, Porto, Portugal.
Santos AI	Rheumatology Department, Hospital Garcia de Orta, Almada, Portugal. filipevinagre@netcabo.pt
Vinagre F	Rheumatology Department, Hospital Garcia de Orta, Almada, Portugal. filipevinagre@netcabo.pt

Serbia

Name of Author	Institutional Affiliation
Damjanov NS	Institute of Rheumatology, Pathology, Social Medicine and Informatics, and Otorhinolaryngology, School of Medicine, University of Belgrade, 11000 Belgrade, Serbia. veramilic@ptt.rs
Milic VD	Institute of Rheumatology, Pathology, Social Medicine and Informatics, and Otorhinolaryngology, School of Medicine, University of Belgrade, 11000 Belgrade, Serbia. veramilic@ptt.rs

Singapore

Name of Author	Institutional Affiliation
Chai J	Department of Neurology, National NeuroScience Institute, Singapore.
Logigian EL	Department of Neurology, National NeuroScience Institute, Singapore.

Spain

Name of Author	Institutional Affiliation
Bosch X	Sjogren Syndrome Research Group (AGAUR), Josep Font Laboratory of Autoimmune Diseases, IDIBAPS, Department of Autoimmune Diseases, Hospital Clinic, C/Villarroel, 170, 08036 Barcelona, Spain. mramos@clinic.ub.es
Coca A	Sjogren Syndrome Research Group (AGAUR), Laboratory of Autoimmune Diseases Josep Font, Institut d'Investigacions Biomediques August Pi i Sunyer, Department of Autoimmune Diseases, Barcelona, Spain.
Davalos A	Neurology Department, Hospital Universitari Germans Trias i Pujol, Badalona, Spain.
Galvez J	Rheumatology Unit, Hospital General Universitario JM Morales Meseguer, C/ Marques de los Velez s/n, Murcia 30008, Spain. ppgalvis@hotmail.com
Marcos M	Department of Autoimmune Diseases, Institut d'Investigacions Biomediques August Pi i Sunyer (IDIBAPS), Hospital Clinic, Barcelona, Spain.
Margaix-Munoz M	Hospital General Universitario, Servicio de Estomatologia, Avda. Tres Cruces s/n, 46014 Valencia, Spain,margaix1980@hotmail.com.
Martinez S	Neurology Department, Hospital Universitari Germans Trias i Pujol, Badalona, Spain.
Perez-De-Lis M	Sjogren Syndrome Research Group (AGAUR), Laboratory of Autoimmune Diseases Josep Font, Institut d'Investigacions Biomediques August Pi i Sunyer, Department of Autoimmune Diseases, Barcelona, Spain.
Pons F	From the Sjogren Syndrome Research Group (AGAUR), Laboratory of Autoimmune Diseases Josep Font, IDIBAPS, Department of Autoimmune Diseases; Nuclear Medicine Department (Centre de Diagnostic per la Imatge); CAP Les Corts, GESCLINIC, Hospital Clinic, Barcelona; and Rheumatology Unit, Hospital 9 d'Octubre, Valencia, Spain.

Ramos-Casals M	Sjogren's Syndrome Research Group (AGAUR), Laboratory of Autoimmune Diseases Josep Font, IDIBAPS, Department of Autoimmune Diseases, Hospital Clinic, Barcelona, Spain. mariajose.soto@uca.es
Reyes Y	Rheumatology Unit, Hospital General Universitario JM Morales Meseguer, C/ Marques de los Velez s/n, Murcia 30008, Spain. ppgalvis@hotmail.com
Sanchez-Tapias JM	Laboratory of Autoimmune Diseases Josep Font, Department of Autoimmune Diseases, Institut d'Investigacions Biomediques August Pi i Sunyer (IDIBAPS), Hospital Clinic, 08036-Barcelona, Spain. mramos@clinic.ub.es
Sarrion G	Hospital General Universitario, Servicio de Estomatologia, Avda. Tres Cruces s/n, 46014 Valencia, Spain,margaix1980@hotmail.com.
Soto-Cardenas MJ	Sjogren's Syndrome Research Group (AGAUR), Laboratory of Autoimmune Diseases Josep Font, IDIBAPS, Department of Autoimmune Diseases, Hospital Clinic, Barcelona, Spain. mariajose.soto@uca.es
Zeron PB	Laboratory of Autoimmune Diseases "Josep Font," IDIBAPS, Department of Autoimmune Diseases, C/Villaroel 170, Hospital Clinic, Barcelona 08036, Spain. mramos@clinic.ub.es

Sweden

Name of Author	Institutional Affiliation
Hammar O	Department of Clinical Sciences, Division of Gastroenterology and Hepatology, Skane University Hospital, Lund University, Malmo, Sweden. oskar.hammar@med.lu.se
Hussein SZ	Department of Rheumatology, Lund University, Skane University Hospital, Malmo, Sweden.
Jacobsson LT	Department of Rheumatology, Malmo University Hospital, Lund University, 20502 Malmo, Sweden. elke.theander@med.lu.se

Mandl T	Department of Rheumatology, Ing 25 plan 2, Malmo University Hospital, S-205 02 Malmo, Sweden. thomas.mandl@med.lu.se
Mannerkorpi K	Department of Rheumatology and Inflammation Research, Sahlgrenska Academy, Goteborg University, Sweden. helena.forsblad@vgregion.se
Theander E	Department of Rheumatology, Malmo University Hospital, Lund University, 20502 Malmo, Sweden. elke.theander@med.lu.se
d'Elia HF	Department of Rheumatology and Inflammation Research, Sahlgrenska Academy, Goteborg University, Sweden. helena.forsblad@vgregion.se

Taiwan

Name of Author	Institutional Affiliation
Kang JH	Department of Physical Medicine and Rehabilitation and Neuroscience Research Center, Taipei, Taiwan.
Lin HC	Department of Physical Medicine and Rehabilitation and Neuroscience Research Center, Taipei, Taiwan.

Turkey

Name of Author	Institutional Affiliation
Gur A	Division of Rheumatology, Department of Physical Medicine and Rehabilitation, Firat University, Faculty of Medicine, Elazig, Turkey. sozgocmen@hotmail.com
Inal V	Division of Rheumatology, Department of Internal Medicine, Ege University School of Medicine, Izmir, Turkey.
Kabasakal Y	Division of Rheumatology, Department of Internal Medicine, Ege University School of Medicine, Izmir, Turkey.
Ozgocmen S	Division of Rheumatology, Department of Physical Medicine and Rehabilitation, Firat University, Faculty of Medicine, Elazig, Turkey. sozgocmen@hotmail.com

Terzioglu E	Division of Rheumatology and Immunology, Department of Internal Medicine, Akdeniz Universitesi Tip Fakultesi Ic Hastaliklari AD, Antalya, Turkey. drvyazisiz@yahoo.com.tr
Toker E	Department of Rheumatology, Marmara University Medical School, Istanbul, Turkey. suleyavuz@gmail.com
Yavuz S	Department of Rheumatology, Marmara University Medical School, Istanbul, Turkey. suleyavuz@gmail.com
Yazisiz V	Division of Rheumatology and Immunology, Department of Internal Medicine, Akdeniz Universitesi Tip Fakultesi Ic Hastaliklari AD, Antalya, Turkey. drvyazisiz@yahoo.com.tr

United Kingdom

Name of Author	Institutional Affiliation
Bourke BE	St George's Hospital, Blackshaw Road, Tooting, London, UK. satishmohanreddy@yahoo.com
Bowman SJ	University of Newcastle, Institute of Cellular Medicine, Musculoskeletal Research Group, Newcastle upon Tyne, NE2 4HH, UK. wan-fai.ng@ncl.ac.uk
Dass S	Academic Unit of Musculoskeletal Disease, University of Leeds, Leeds, UK.
Emery P	Academic Unit of Musculoskeletal Disease, University of Leeds, Leeds, UK.
Fedele S	UCL Eastman Dental Institute, London, United Kingdom. s.fedele@eastman.ucl.ac.uk
Kamel UF	North West Wales NHS Trust, Bangor University, Bangor, UK.
Konttinen YT	UCL Eastman Dental Institute, London, United Kingdom. s.fedele@eastman.ucl.ac.uk
Ng WF	University of Newcastle, Institute of Cellular Medicine, Musculoskeletal Research Group, Newcastle upon Tyne, NE2 4HH, UK. wan-fai.ng@ncl.ac.uk
Rachapalli SM	St George's Hospital, Blackshaw Road, Tooting, London, UK. satishmohanreddy@yahoo.com

Rauz S	Department of Rheumatology, University Hospital Birmingham NHS Foundation Trust (Selly Oak), Raddlebarn Road, Birmingham B296JD, UK. simon.bowman@uhb.nhs.uk
Whitaker R	North West Wales NHS Trust, Bangor University, Bangor, UK.

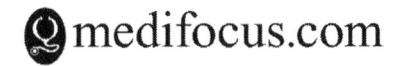

NOTES

Use this page for taking notes as you review your Guidebook

5 - Tips on Finding and Choosing a Doctor

Introduction

One of the most important decisions confronting patients who have been diagnosed with a serious medical condition is finding and choosing a qualified physician who will deliver a high level and quality of medical care in accordance with currently accepted guidelines and standards of care. Finding the "best" doctor to manage your condition, however, can be a frustrating and time-consuming experience unless you know what you are looking for and how to go about finding it.

The process of finding and choosing a physician to manage your specific illness or condition is, in some respects, analogous to the process of making a decision about whether or not to invest in a particular stock or mutual fund. After all, you wouldn't invest your hard eared money in a stock or mutual fund without first doing exhaustive research about the stock or fund's past performance, current financial status, and projected future earnings. More than likely you would spend a considerable amount of time and energy doing your own research and consulting with your stock broker before making an informed decision about investing. The same general principle applies to the process of finding and choosing a physician. Although the process requires a considerable investment in terms of both time and energy, the potential payoff can be well worth it--after all, what can be more important than your health and well-being?

This section of your Guidebook offers important tips for how to find physicians as well as suggestions for how to make informed choices about choosing a doctor who is right for you.

Tips for Finding Physicians

Finding a highly qualified, competent, and compassionate physician to manage your specific illness or condition takes a lot of hard work and energy but is an investment that is well-worth the effort. It is important to keep in mind that you are not looking for just any general physician but rather for a physician who has expertise in the treatment and management of your specific illness or condition. Here are some suggestions for where you can turn to identify and locate physicians who specialize in managing your disorder:

- **Your Doctor** - Your family physician (family medicine or internal medicine specialist) is a good starting point for finding a physician who specializes in your illness. Chances are that your doctor already knows several specialists in your geographic area who specialize in your illness and can recommend several names to you. Your doctor can also provide you with information about their qualifications, training, and hospital affiliations.

- **Your Peer Network** - Your family, friends, and co-workers can be a potentially very useful network for helping you find a physician who specializes in your illness. They may know someone else with this condition and may be able to put you in touch with them to find out which doctors they can recommend. If you have friends, neighbors, or relatives who work in hospitals (e.g., nurses, social workers, administrators), they may be a potentially valuable source for helping you find a physician who specializes in your condition.

- **Hospitals and Medical Centers** - Hospitals and medical centers are, potentially, an excellent source for finding physicians who specialize in treating specific diseases. Simply contact hospitals and major medical centers in your city, county, or state and ask if they have anyone on their staff who specializes in treating your condition. When you call, ask to speak to someone in the specific Department that cares for patients with the illness. For example, if you have been diagnosed with cancer, ask to speak with someone in the Department of Hematology and Oncology. If you are not sure which Department treats patients with your specific condition, ask to speak to someone in the Department of Medicine since this Department is the umbrella for many other medical specialties.

- **Organizations and Support Groups** - Many disease organizations and support groups that cater to patients with a specific illness or condition maintain physician referral lists and may be able to recommend doctors in your geographic area who specialize in the treatment and management of your specific disorder. This *MediFocus Guidebook* includes a select listing of disease organizations and support groups that you may wish to contact to ask for a physician referral.

- **Managed Care Plans** - If you belong to a managed care plan, you can obtain a list of physicians who belong to the Plan from the plan's membership services office. Keep in mind, however, that your choices will usually be limited to only those doctors who belong to the Plan. If you decide to go outside the Plan, you will likely have to pay for the doctor's services "out of pocket".

- **Medical Journals** - Many doctors based at major medical centers and universities who have special interest in a particular disease or condition conduct research and publish their findings in leading medical journals. Searching the medical literature can help you identify and locate leading physicians who are recognized as experts in their field about a particular illness. This *MediFocus Guidebook* includes an extensive listing of the names and institutional affiliations of physicians and researchers, in the United States and other countries, who have recently published their studies about this specific medical condition in leading medical journals. You can also conduct your own online search for your illness or condition and identify additional authors and hospitals who specialize in the disease using the PubMed database available at http://www.nlm.nih.gov.

- **American Medical Association** - The American Medical Association (AMA) is the nation's largest professional medical association that represents many doctors in the United States and also provides a free physician locator service called "AMA Physician Select" available at http://dbapps.ama-assn.org/aps/amahg.htm. You can search the AMA database by either "Physician Name" or "Medical Specialty". You can find information about physicians including medical school and residency training, area of specialty, and contact information.

- **American Board of Medical Specialists** - The American Board of Medical Specialists (ABMS) publishes a geographical list of board-certified physicians called the Official ABMS Directory of Board Certified Medical Specialists that is available in most public libraries. Physicians who are listed in the ABMS Directory are board-certified in a medical specialty meaning that they have passed rigorous certification examinations administered by a board of medical specialists. There are 24 specialty boards that are recognized by the ABMS and the AMA. Each candidate applying for board certification must pass a written examination given by the specific specialty board and 15 of the specialty boards also require candidates to pass an oral examination in order to obtain board certification. To find out if a particular physician you are considering is board certified:

  - Visit your local public library and ask for a copy of the Official ABMS Directory of Board Certified Medical Specialists.

  - Search the ABMS web site at http://www.abms.org/login.asp.

  - Call the ABMS toll free at 1-866-275-2267.

- **American Society of Clinical Oncology** - The American Society of Clinical Onclology (ASC)) is the largest professional organization that represents physicians who specialize in treating cancer patients (oncologists). The ASCO provides a searchable database of ASCO members called "Find an Oncologist" that you can access online at http://www.asco.org. You can search the "Find an Oncologist" database for a cancer specialist by name, city, state, country, or specialty area.

- **American Cancer Society** - The American Cancer Society (ACS) is a nationwide voluntary health organization dedicated to helping cancer patients and survivors through research, education, advocacy, and services. The ACS web site http://www.cancer.org is not only an excellent resource for cancer information but also includes a "Message Board" where you can ask questions, exchange ideas, and share stories. The ACS Message Board is also a potentially useful source for locating an oncologist in your geographical area who specializes in your specific type of cancer. You can also contact the ACS toll free by calling 1-800-ACS-2345.

- **National Comprehensive Cancer Network** - The National Comprehensive Cancer Network (NCCN) is an alliance of 19 of the world's leading cancer centers and is dedicated to helping patients and health care professionals make informed decisions about cancer care. You can find a listing of the 19 NCCN member cancer institutions on the NCCN web site at http://www.nccn.org/. You can also search the NCCN "Physician Directory" for doctors located at any of the 19 NCCN member cancer institutions at http://www.nccn.org/physician_directory/SearchPers.asp. This database is an excellent resource for locating leading cancer specialists nationwide who specialize in your specific type of cancer.

- **National Cancer Institute Clinical Trials Database** - The National Cancer Institute (NCI) is part of the National Institutes of Health (NIH) and coordinates the National Cancer Program which conducts and supports research, training, and a variety of other programs dedicated to prevention and treatment of cancer. The NCI maintains an extensive cancer clinical trials database that you can access at http://www.cancer.gov/clinicaltrials. You can search the database for current clinical trials by type of cancer and even limit your search to clinical trials within you geographical area by putting in your Zip Code. The NCI clinical trials database also provides contact information for the physicians who serve as the study coordinators for each clinical trial. This database is a valuable resource for identifying and locating leading physicians in your local area and around the country who are conducting cutting-edge clinical research about your specific type of cancer.

- **National Center for Complementary and Alternative Medicine** - The National Center for Complementary and Alternative Medicine (NCCAM) is part of the National Institutes of Health (NIH) and is dedicated to exploring complementary and alternative medicine healing practices in the context of rigorous scientific research and methodology. The NCCAM web site http://nccam.nih.gov/ includes publications, frequently asked questions, and useful links to other complementary and alternative medicine resources. If you have questions about complementary and alternative medicine practices for your particular illness or medical condition, you can contact the NCCAM Clearinghouse toll-free in the U.S. at 1-888-644-6226 or 301-519-3153. You can also contact the NCCAM Clearinghouse by E-mail: info@nccam.nih.gov.

- **National Organization for Rare Disorders** - The National Organization for Rare Disorders (NORD) is a federation of voluntary health organizations dedicated to helping patients with rare "orphan" diseases and their families. There are over 6,000 rare or "orphan" diseases that are estimated to affect approximately 25 million Americans. You can search NORD's "Rare Diseases Database" for information about rare diseases at http://www.rarediseases.org/search/rdblist.html. In addition to providing useful information about rare diseases, NORD maintains a confidential "Networking Program" for its members to enable them to communicate with other patients who suffer from the same disorder. To learn more about NORD's Networking Program, you can send an E mail to: orphan@rarediseases.org.

How to Make Informed Choices About Physicians

It has generally been assumed by many people that the longer a physician has been in practice, the more experience, knowledge, and skills he/she has accumulated and, therefore, the higher the quality of care they provide to their patients. Recent research conducted by a group of doctors from the Harvard Medical School, however, seems to strongly suggest that this premise may not be true. In an article published in February 2005 in the *Annals of Internal Medicine* (Volume 142, No. 4, pp. 260-303), the Harvard researchers seriously challenged the common assumption that the more clinical experience a physician has accumulated, the higher the level of medical care they provide to their patients.

In fact, surprisingly, the researchers found an inverse (opposite) relationship between the number of years that a physician has been in practice (i.e., experience) and the quality of care that the physician provides. In other words, the widely held belief that "practice makes perfect" does not necessarily apply to all physicians and should not be the sole criteria used by patients in their decision analysis for choosing a physician. The underlying message of this study is that the length of time a physician has been in practice does not necessarily equate to a high quality of medical care unless the doctor takes steps to keep abreast with new advances and changing patterns of clinical practice.

Here are some important issues you need to consider and carefully research before making an informed decision about choosing your doctor:

- **Board Certification** - Board certified doctors are required to have extra training after medical school to become specialists in a particular field of medicine and are required to take continuing education courses in order to maintain their board certification status. Check with the American Board of Medical Specialists (ABMS) to determine if a specific physician you are considering is board certified in a particular medical specialty. To find out if a particular physician you are considering is board certified:

    - Visit your local public library and ask for a copy of the Official ABMS Directory of Board Certified Medical Specialists.

    - Search the ABMS web site at http://www.abms.org/login.asp.

    - Call the ABMS toll free at 1-866-275-2267.

- **Experience** - As noted above, research from the Harvard Medical School strongly suggests that how long a physician has been in practice (i.e., experience) does not necessarily correlate with a high level of medical care. The most important issue, therefore, is not how long a doctor has been in practice but rather how much experience the physician has in treating your specific illness or medical condition. Some physicians who have been in practice for many decades may have only treated a small number of patients with the specific disorder, whereas, some younger physicians who have been in practice only a few years may have already treated hundreds of patients with the same disorder. Here are some suggestions for helping you find out about a particular physician's experience in treating your specific illness:

    - Call the physician's office and speak with a staff member such as a nurse or physician's assistant. Ask them for information about how many patients with your specific medical condition the physician treats during the course of a year. Ask how many patients with this condition the physician is currently treating. You will have to call several different physicians' offices in order to have a basis for comparing the numbers of patients.

    - Find out if the physician has published any articles about the condition in reputable medical journals by doing an author search online. You can conduct an online author search using PubMed at http://www.nlm.nih.gov. Simply click on the "PubMed" icon, select the "author" field from the "Limits" menu, enter the physician's name (last name followed by first initial), and then click on the "Go" button. The author search will retrieve all articles published by the particular physician you are considering.

- Talk with your family physician and ask if he/she can provide you with any information about the particular physician's experience in treating patients with your specific illness or condition.

- Contact disease organizations and support groups that specialize in helping patients with your specific disorder and ask if they can provide you with any information, including experience, about the physician you are considering.

- **Medical School Affiliation** - Find out if the physician you are considering also has a joint faculty appointment at a medical school. In general, practicing community physicians with a joint academic appointment at a medical school are more likely to be in contact with leading medical experts and may be more up-to-date with the latest advances in research and treatments than community based physicians who are not affiliated with a medical school.

- **Hospital Affiliation** - Find out about the hospitals that the doctor uses. In the event that you need to be treated at a hospital, is the hospital where the physician has admitting privileges nearby to your home or will you (and your family members) have to travel a considerable distance?

- **Hospital Accreditation** - Find out if the hospital where the physician has admitting privileges is accredited by the Joint Commission on Accreditation of Healthcare Organizations (JCAHO). You can find information about a specific hospital's accreditation status by searching the JCAHO web site at http://www.jointcommission.org/. The JCAHO is an independent, not-for-profit organization that evaluates and accredits more than 15,000 health care organizations and programs in the United States. To receive and maintain JCAHO accreditation, a health care organization must undergo an on-site survey by a JCAHO survey team at least every three years and meet specific standards and performance measurements that affect the safety and quality of patient care.

- **Health Insurance Coverage** - Find out if the physician is covered by your health insurance plan. If you belong to a managed care plan (HMO or PPO), you are usually restricted to using specific physicians who also belong to the Plan. If you decide to use a physician who is "outside the network," you will likely have to pay "out of pocket" for the services provided.

NOTES

Use this page for taking notes as you review your Guidebook

6 - Directory of Organizations

American Academy of Ophthalmology
POB 7424; San Francisco, CA 94120-7424
415.561.8500
customer_service@aao.org
www.aao.org

American Autoimmune Related Diseases Association
22100 Gratiot Avenue; E. Detroit, MI 48021
800.598.4668; 586.776.3900
www.aarda.org

American College of Rheumatology
1800 Century Place; Suite 250; Atlanta, GA 30345-4300
404.633.3777
acr@rheumatology.org
www.rheumatology.org

Arthritis Foundation
POB 7669; Atlanta, GA 30309
800.283.7800
arthritisfoundation@arthritis.org
www.arthritis.org

British Sjogren's Syndrome Association
PO Box 10867 Birmingham B16 0ZW UK
01214556532
office@bssa.uk.net
www.bssa.uk.net/

Dry.org
dry.org

Johns Hopkins Arthritis Center
5501 Hopkins Bayview Circle Asthma and Allergy Center Floor 1B Baltimore, Maryland 21224
410.550.8089
jhuarthritis@jhmi.edu
www.hopkins-arthritis.org/

National Institute of Arthritis and Musculoskeletal; and Skin Diseases Information Clearinghouse
National Institutes of Health; 1 AMS Circle; Bethesda, MD 20892-3675
301.495.4484; 877.226.4267; 301.565.2966 (TTY)
niamsinfo@mail.nih.gov
www.niams.nih.gov

National Organization for Rare Disorders
P.O. Box 1968 (55 Kenosia Avenue) Danbury, CT   06813-1968
800-999-NORD (6673)
orphan@rarediseases.org
www.rarediseases.org

Sjogren's World
sjogrens@sjogrensworld.org
www.sjsworld.org

Sjogren's Syndrome Genetics Studies; University of Minnesota; Sjogren's Study
5-150 MCB Bldg.; 420 Washington Avenue; Minneapolis, MN 55455
612.624.5922
info@sjogrensgenes.org
biosips.org/

medifocus.com

Sjogren's Syndrome Foundation
6707 Democracy Blvd. Suite 325 Bethesda, MD 20817
301.530.4420; 800.475.6473
www.sjogrens.com

Complementary and Alternative Medicine Resources

American Academy of Medical Acupuncture
170 East Grand Avenue Suite 330 El Segundo, CA 90245 Phone: 310.364.0193
administrato@medicalacupuncture.org
http://www.medicalacupuncture.org

American Association for Acupuncture and Oriental Medicine
1925 West County Road B2
Roseville, MN 55113
Phone: 651.631.0216
http://www.aaaom.edu

American Association of Naturopathic Physicians
4435 Wisconsin Avenue
Suite 403 Washington, DC 20016
Phone (Toll free): 866.538.2267
Phone: 202.237.8150
http://www.naturopathic.org

American Chiropractic Association
1701 Clarendon Blvd.
Arlington, VA 22209
Phone: 703.276.8800 memberinfo@acatoday.org http://www.amerchiro.org

American Holistic Medical Association
23366 Commerce Park Suite 101B Beachwood, OH 44122 Phone: 216.292.6644
info@holisticmedicine.org http://www.holisticmedicine.org

American Massage Therapy Association
500 Davis Street, Suite 900
Evanston, IL 60201-4695
Phone (Toll-Free): 877.905.2700
Phone: 847.864.0123 info@amtamassage.org http://www.amtamassage.org

National Center for Complementary and Alternative Medicine (NCCAM) Clearinghouse
9000 Rockville Pike Bethesda, MD 20892 Phone: 888.644.6226 info@nccam.nih.gov

http://nccam.nih.gov

National Center for Homeopathy
801 North Fairfax Street, Suite 306
Alexandria, VA 22314
Phone: 703.548.7790
http://www.homeopathic.org

Office of Dietary Supplements, National Institutes of Health
6100 Executive Boulevard
Room 3B01, MSC 7517
Bethesda, MD 20892-7517
Phone: 301.435.2920   ods@nih.gov   http://ods.od.nih.gov

Rosenthal Center for Complementary and Alternative Medicine
Columbia Presbyterian Hospital
630 West 168th Street
Box 75
New York, NY 10032
Phone: 212.342.0101
http://rosenthal.hs.columbia.edu

Made in the USA
Charleston, SC
23 May 2012